DIY
Organic Medications

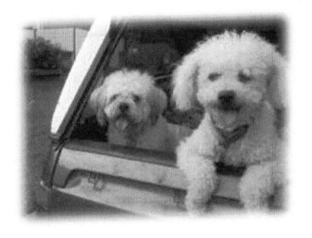

Aromatherapy based cures in this book, suit most animals and all humans.

Author

Robyna Smith- Keys

This Book

Dog Care & DIY Organic Medications

ISBN-13: 978-1974439317
ISBN-10: 1974439313

Published by Robyna Smith-Keys
Beauty School Books
Reedy Creek . Queensland
Australia 4227
www.beautyschollbooks.com

Introduction

Before you begin it is significantly important, that you read the entire section on "Aromatherapy for Dogs" and all sub headings under Aromatherapy.

As a trained Aromatherapist with two darling white fluffy dogs I often self medicate my dogs. Mark Antony pictured on the right is a Bechon Frise, he is thirteen in October 2013. Ceasar his son is half Maltese and half Bechon Frise. Ceasar will be nine in May 2013; Ceasar is pictured on the left. They are living proof that what I have tried, works.

There are many times and an enormous amount of reasons why people cannot go to a Veterinary surgeon. It is my hope with this book to assist you with lowering the cost of pet-care and save you from those anxious moments. After all they are our most loyal friends. However, I find caring for dogs is more challenging than caring for children.

Prevention is always better than a cure. Learn all there is to know about your dog. I check my dog gums every morning before they have their morning treat.

Dog Care & DIY Organic Medication

Before purchasing this book please note, I can only help you with minor ailments, flea infestation and minor accidents. For all major accidents or illnesses, you will still require the services of a Veterinarian. The abbreviation for Veterinarian throughout this book is "Vet"

Book Contents

Aromatherapy for Dogs

Aromatherapy Is The Earths Healer.

This book is about dogs but aromatherapy can be used to heal humans and all kinds of animals and creatures.

Liquids are extracted from plants, leaves, flowers and roots. Theses liquids are called "Essential Oils". To produce 1 kilogram of Rose oil you need to extract by steam distillation around 10 acres of Rose leaves. This makes essential oils very expensive; however you may purchase Essential oils in 5-10 ml bottles from around $9. Please do not purchase fragrance oils as they are a synthetic liquid. Fragrance oils cannot, be used for healing purposes. In France Doctors will made Essential oils into a medicine but in Australia the Therapeutic Goods Association insists that essential oils may only be used as a topical medication and are a "Nil By Mouth" medication.

Essential Oils Are:

- Dynamic vegetable hormones
- A liquid not an oil
- A nil by mouth therapeutic substance
- An additive for massage oils and other therapeutic treatments

What Most Essential Oils Have In Common:-

- Anti-bacterial, anti-microbic, anti-virus properties

- Detoxify - gets rid of poisons from our blood stream. (Urine is usually pale yellow, as it gets darker; it is a sign of toxins being discarded)

- Oxygenate - as oxygen is added to our body it has the effect of pumping up the tissues, so does exercise such as Yoga

- Temporarily helps rid tissues of excess fluid

Essential oils are easily absorbed by the skin because they are lipo-solvents - they dissolve in fats. They dissolve in the fatty part of the skin to quickly penetrate different layers before entering the bloodstream (Sebaceous glands produce Seba, the Essential oils blend with the Seba and makes for easy absorption).

It is important to understand a few Aromatherapy safety rules before you start using Essential Oils for healing. You would perhaps give a sick adult two Aspirin or Aspros if they had the flue but you would not give the same dose to a small child. Throughout this book, I have given recipes for different ailments. It takes four years to complete an Aromatherapy degree and a lifetime of learning to become proficient at healing with Essential oils.

It is not my intension with this book, to neither baffle you with science nor scare you into being too afraid not to try self-medicating your best friend (your dog).

Keep it simple, stick strictly to the recipe and administer the treatment with love.

1) Some Essential Oils such as Rosemary can be lethal to some people and very healing in a small dose to other people.

2) Essential Oils are very strong and should never ever be used straight from the bottle. They must always be added to a base oil or fatty substance such as butter or cream.

You must not take it upon yourself to add extra oils. You must read all my section on Aromatherapy blending and mixing along with the "Oils To Be Avoided" section than Bobs your uncle.

How To Heal With Aromatherapy:-

 I trust there is enough info here for you not to need to buy any other book. However you will find loads of more information about illnesses, complaints, and ailment under the A-Z headings.

Note: this section can be found in my Aromatherapy books. A good basic book is my book called "Foolproof Aromatherapy". Pick 1-3 (no more than 3) essential oil from the appropriate ailments list, mix 1-3 essential oil with 100 ml of carrier oil.

Massage into the effected region. Always mix the essential oils with 100 ml of carrier oil. Only use cold pressed Olive oil, Grape seed, Jojoba or Almond oil.

Check and double check the "Oils To Be Avoided" section.

Note: These strengths are for adults only and 50 drops of Essential oils are for the body not the face. When mixing for the face only use half the amount of essential oil that you would use on the body. Never massage yourself any more than 4 times a week and never apply any of the mixtures below more than twice a day for 4 days unless otherwise stated.

For animals never use more than twice a day for three days, unless the recipe states otherwise. Give the animal two days without treatment of essential oils then resume treatment for another three days.

Aromatherapy Blending Chart

This is a typical blending chart for humans. The dose you use on dogs is the same does that you would use on babies over nine months. However, I use the same mix as for children but as you are not trained in the contra-indications please use the recipes I have provided or mix for babies.

First, you look up in the "Oils To Be Avoided Chart" which oils not to use under certain conditions. Then you would look up the ailment in the A-Z list. For example a spider bite would be listed under "B" for bites, it may also have a listing under "S" that would say see bites. I have tried to use recipes that are safe in all situations but it is a good idea if your pet has a heart condition or takes fits to check on the "Oils to be avoided section".

As stated earlier in this book Essential oils should, never be applied directly onto the skin nor should they be mixed with food or other products.

Mixing For Adults

Adult Body
100 ml of carrier oil add 50 drops of Essential oil
50 ml of carrier oil add 25 drops of Essential oil
6 ml of carrier oil add 3 drops of Essential oil

Adult Face
100 ml of carrier oil add 25 drops of Essential oil
50 ml of carrier oil add 12.5 drops of Essential oil
6 ml of carrier oil add 1 drops of Essential oil

Children

Children over 5 and under 12 years use the same mixture as for the adult face.

Pregnancy

Pregnancy only after the 1st trimester and only use the oils allowed as per the page headed Pregnancy.

Animal Pregnancy

For very small and medium size animals avoid using essential oil until the animal has labor pains. For large sized animals like a horse, giraffe, elephant use half the does as prescribed here and never during the first eight weeks of the pregnancy.

100 ml of carrier oil add 6 drops of Essential oil
50 ml of carrier oil add 4 drops of Essential oil

Babies & Puppies

Babies never ever until 6 months old and never without an Aromatherapist consultation.

Babies Over One Year Old To Five Years

100 ml of carrier oil add 3- 5 drops of Essential oil
50 ml of carrier oil add 1 - 2 drops of Essential oil
25 ml of carrier oil add 1 drops of Essential oil

Animals Over 30 Kilo (Not Pregnant)

100 ml of carrier oil add 10 drops of Essential oil
50 ml of carrier oil add 5 drops of Essential oil
 6 ml of carrier oil add 1 drops of Essential oil

Essential oils must only, be placed in either food safe plastic or a dark coloured glass bottle. Glass should always be your first choice. If you do not have a dark coloured bottle, you can use a clear clean glass bottle or jar and keep it in a brown paper bag. Light spoils oil and will turn it into a toxin. Air also spoils oil so keep the lid on tight. Also, replace the lid immediately after opening.

Aromatherapy Safe Essential Oils

Safe essential oils: The following Essential Oils are considered safe and acceptable when used correctly. Never use straight from the bottle in its full strength always mix with carrier oil. Always check "The Oils To Be Avoided" list.

Nil by mouth.

- Angelica
- Aniseed
- Basil
- Bay
- Benzoin
- Bergamot
- Black Pepper
- Caraway Seed
- Cardamom
- Carrot Seed
- Cascarilla
- Cedar-wood
- Cinnamon Leaf
- Clary Sage
- Coriander
- Cypress
- Everlasting
- Fennel (Sweet)
- Frankincense
- Galbanum
- Geranium
- Ginger

- Hyssop
- Jasmine
- Lemongrass
- Marjoram (French Type)
- Melissa
- Myrrh
- Neroli
- Nutmeg
- Rose Geranium
- Origanum
- Palmarosa
- Parsley seed
- Patchouli
- Peppermint
- Petitgrain
- Pine
- Rose and Rose Geranium
- Rosewood
- Sage
- Sandalwood
- Verbena
- Vetiver
- Violet Leaf
- Yarrow
- Ylang Ylang

Oils To Be Avoided

Oils to be avoided under certain conditions:-

Antidote To Homeopathy Remedies:

- Black Pepper
- Eucalyptus
- Peppermint
- White Camphor

High Blood Pressure

(Hypertension per = high) Do not use:-
- Basil
- Eucalyptus (all)
- Peppermint
- Rosemary
- Thyme (all varieties),
- Sage

Low Blood Pressure

(Hypotension po=low) Do not use:-

- Clary Sage
- Lavender
- Lemon
- Melissa
- Marjoram,
- Ylang Ylang

Photosensitive to most skin types:-

Note all of these oils are in the safe to use list but they are not safe if you are going to the beach or out to play in the sun as they will cause brown sport on the skin like very large freckles.

- Angelica
- Bergamot
- Grapefruit

- Lemon
- Lemongrass
- Lime
- Mandarin
- Orange
- Tangerine
- Verbena

Photo toxic:

(Do not use during the day, go into sun or under a sun lamp)

- Bergamot,
- Lemon
- Orange
- Neroli

When I am going into the sun, I never use any of the Photosensitive/ Photo Toxic oils and the same rule should apply for your animals. They will cause burning to the deeper layers of the skin cells. It is best to apply photosensitive oils in the evening to yourself or to your animals.

Animals:- Not until they are three months old. Unless prescribed by an Aromatherapist.

Then follow the same blending table as for children. For small dogs and cats that are less than 15 kilo (33 pounds) follow the mixing instructions for Babies.

Babies not at all under six months

See section headed "Baby Oils" that are safest for 6 month old to 2 years: Note more info, can be found in my Aromatherapy books.

- German- Chamomile,
- Lavender
- Mandarin
- (But in a 1/2% dilution for massage) and only one drop in a bath with 2 - 3 tablespoons of carrier.

Unsafe For Lactation

Oils that interfere or dry up milk flow during Lactation:
- Clary Sage
- Peppermint
- Sage (blocks the milk duct)

- Safe Oils For Lactation:
- Lemongrass,
- Geranium
- Fennel (1/2%-1%) but diluted

Oils That Irritate Skin

Oils That Can Cause Skin Sensitization Or Irritate

A Sensitive Skin Type:-

- Basil
- Cedarwood
- Cypress
- Eucalyptus
- Fennel
- Lemon
- Lemongrass
- Lime
- Peppermint
- Pine
- Tea Tree
- Thyme

- Ylang Ylang.

It does upset me somewhat that people think it is safe to use Tea Tree oil on your face because it dries up pimples and puss. Which is true, but what they do not tell you is, it dries up your sebaceous glands as well. Have a read of this info:-

https://www.theguardian.com/science/2007/feb/18/medicineand health.health

Oils Not To Use For: Inhalations, Douches, Enemas:

Thyme (all varieties) never use thyme ever.

Oils That Are Mucous Membrane Irritants:

Cajuput (comes from the Tea Tree family)
Thyme,

Oils Not To Be Used While Pregnant.

Oils That Have Emmenagogue Properties (i.e. promotes menstrual flow):
Massage can commence after the first trimester, after client has been to the doctors to check all health aspects.

Animals only massage the animal in the evening and only with a mixture of 50 ml Olive oil and one drop of Chamomile. Keep this mixture in a dark glass bottle.

Never Use Any Of These Oils While Pregnant:-

- Basil,
- Cedar-wood
- Fennel,
- Clary Sage,
- Myrrh
- Marjoram
- Peppermint
- Sage
- Thyme.

These constituents affect the liver by making it overwork in order to excrete them. Robert Tisser states that 65% of the convulsive essential oils contain ketone constituents, and six out of eight of the abortifacient essential oils, so caution is needed.

Safest Essential Oils To Use In Pregnancy:

- Chamomile (German),
- Lavender,
- Neroli,
- Orange,
- Tangerine,
- Mandarin,
- Lemon,
- Sandalwood,
- Rosewood.
- Epilepsy

The oils that are convulsive or can cause epilepsy are generally made up of Phenols or Oxides which in large dosages can cause convulsions and be neuro-toxic, so correct dosages are important when blending. Phenols are the most irritant on skin and mucous membranes and they can damage liver if used in massive dosages.

Avoid When Convulsive or Epileptic:-

- Basil
- Eucalyptus (Globulus, Radiata & Polybractea)
- Fennel
- Peppermint
- Rosemary
- Sage
- Thyme

Aromatherapy- is an amazing healer and will surpass most medication, from a Chemist. Essential oils when mixed correctly for the ailment will actual heal where most other forms of medication only suppress the ailment and give the body time to heal itself. However, they are in most cases a slow form of healing.

Pain Releif

A Veterinarian Nurse - told me they give dogs Tamil. The issue I have with Tamil tables is my dogs cough it back up and chew it. That causes other problems as Tamil need to be taken without chewing.

Asprin/Aspro

Never use Aspin unless there is no other option. Aspirin also reduces inflammation. Researchers believe these effects come about because aspirin blocks the production of pain-producing chemicals called prostaglandins.

In addition to relieving pain and reducing inflammation, aspirin also lowers fever by acting on the part of the brain that regulates temperature. The brain then signals the blood vessels to widen, which allows heat to leave the body more quickly. I like to add the occasional pinch of turmeric powder to their food.

Precautions:

Aspirin-even children's aspirin-should never be given to children or teenagers with flu-like symptoms or chickenpox. So the same can be said, for your young animals. In some individuals, Aspirin can cause Reye's syndrome, a life-threatening condition that affects the nervous system and liver. Up to 30% of children and teenagers, who develop Reye's syndrome, die. Those who survive may have permanent brain damage. Reye-like illnesses are most likely to occur in infants under 4 years of age, which may be due to an inherited metabolic disorder.

Check with a physician before giving aspirin to a child under 12 years for arthritis, rheumatism, or any condition that requires long-term use of the drug.

No one should take aspirin for more than 10 days in a row unless told to do so by a physician. Anyone with a fever, should not take aspirin for more than 3 days without a physician's consent. Do not take more than the recommended daily dosage.

I have administered Aspro to my dogs in very small does and my children without adverse results. But, to err on the side of caution and good judgment is strongly recommended.

Remember this book is about helping you when you cannot get to the Veterinary. It is not about replacing a Veterinary that has had at least studied for four years and has many years experience with animals.

Due to the fact that we medicate dogs with the same dose we medicate our Babies use Aspirin/Aspro very sparingly. Never use a slow release type, unless you are able to push straight down their throat without them chewing it. I am not saying to give a baby Asprin/Apro I am saying to treat dogs with the same tiny amount of medication that we give babies. Note: we do not give babies Asprin/Aspro unless a Doctor has recommended it and even them be skeptical.

Fragrance oils

Fragrance oils that are used in burners are not my idea of safe Aromas, and should never be applied to the skin. The cost of these in Australia is around $1.50 - $3.50. You get what you pay for. They are not ideal for fragrance or oil burners either as they emit (send out) toxins into the air.

Fear of Storms

We always know a storm is coming as my daughters 7 year old dog, runs and put her face under the pillow and shades uncontrollably.

This is what I do for her.

I put one drop of Lavender on the pillow.

In one tablespoon of olive oil I add one drop essential oil of lavender. Then I massage this into her stomach. Instantly she stops shaking.

Arthritis

If you follow my feeding and walking instructions, your dogs probably will not get Arthritis. Just like humans, there should not be any wheat, dairy or preservatives in the food your dog consumes.

If your dog has arthritis in the early stages this is what you can do.

First Change His Diet.

Brush him every day for at least ten minutes. Twice a day is better. Use a large bristle hairbrush. Brush towards the heart in a gentle motion followed with a gentle stroking motion with the other hand. As you brush and stroke his shoulders do so in a rotating circular type of stroke.

Wet a thick hand towel, ring it out, roll it up and place in the microwave oven for 30 seconds. Test that it is not burning hot on your own skin near your wrist before applying to your dog. Press this onto his joints and hold for a few minutes.

Apply the Aromatherapy Arthritis mix to all his joints such as his ankle joints, knee and hip joints and to his neck. Then apply heat to each joint for a few minutes.

Heat can be applied in several ways.

- Hot porridge
- Wheat bags
- Rice bags
- Hot towels
- Hot porridge compress

Hot porridge makes a good compress I use it when I have a headache. For your dog, mix porridge with boiling water. Usually half a cup of porridge mixed with a cup of boiling water is a good mix. Place in paper towel and tie to his joints. Or place inside a sock and tie to his affected area.

Wheat Bags

Half fill a small cot pillowslip with wheat and sew the open end so it is completely sealed. Place the wheat slip into the microwave for three minutes on high. Tie the wheat slip with a cotton bandage over the dog's rump for about 5 minutes. Then tie the wheat slip around his back leg for three minutes. Reheat the bag for two minutes in the microwave and tie the wheat slip around his other leg. Repeat this heat treatment for the other three legs.

Rice Bags

I prefer to use rice rather than wheat. When you fill a bag or sock with rice you can add some dried cloves or cardamom pods.

Rice bags have two purposes.

1. They can be heated for a minute or two in the microwave and used as a heat pack for nagging pain

2. Rice bags can be placed in the freezer for acute pain.

Compress Application Hot-Cold

HOT

Hot compresses will ease the pain of these conditions.

- Abscesses
- Backache
- Chest pains of nervous origin
- Chronic pain
- Cramps
- Lumbago/sciatica
- Menstrual cramps
- Muscular aches/pains
- Neuralgia
- Oedema
- Toothache

COLD

Acute pain is often caused by swelling and inflammation. That is when a cold compress or poultice woks its magic.

- Burns
- Contusions
- Fevers
- Fractures (don't massage)
- Headaches
- High Temperatures
- Sprains (Ice)

Heat Bag Socks

You can half fill large football socks with wheat and sew the tops of the socks closed or tie the tops of the socks with string. Do not put too much wheat in the socks, as you will need to wrap the socks around his legs and then put another pair of socks over his legs to keep the wheat socks in place. The socks are best if made of cotton or wool. Socks made from synthetic materials cannot, be used. They will probably burn and cause a fire in the microwave.

When you place the dogs, wheat bags in the microwave be sure to sit in a heatproof bowl so you are not filling your microwave with germs. Then clean the microwave with paper towel and vinegar.

Pain Relief With Ice

No matter if it's a human or animal ice packs are an amazing relief. Some forms of arthritis causes swelling in the joints. It is best to place an ice pack on the swollen area.

Arthritis Mix For Dogs

Dogs 3 to 15 kilograms of body weight.

In 100 ml Olive Oil
Add 2 drops Essential oils of Lavender
2 drops Eucalyptus
1 drop Thyme
2 drops Lemon.

Dogs over 15 kilograms

In 100 ml Olive Oil
Add 2 drops Essential oils of Lavender
5 drops Eucalyptus
1 drop Thyme
4 drops Lemon.

Massage this into his joints each morning.
Less is best. Please do not add more Essential oils than prescribed.

Warning: If your dog has a bad or weak heart condition, do not add Thyme.

In the evening give him a quarter (1/4) of a baby Aspin or Aspro/Aspirin with his food. For small dogs under 10 kilo use one eighth of an Aspro.

Dogs 11 – 25 kilo give quarter of an Aspro

Larger dogs 30-60 kilo a half of an Aspro.

If your dog likes liver treats, wet the treat a little and smear the crushes Aspirin/Aspro onto one side of the liver treat. Fold the treat in half and give to the dog. You can also add to his food or crush and mix with a little honey.

If your dog has arthritis it is very important not to feed him neither dog biscuits nor tin foods that are filled with preservatives and wheat. Keep his food very natural. Steamed meat or chicken with vegetables is all he should have. Twice a week add a pinch of Kelp powder or a few drops of Salmon oil. Plus a pinch of Spirulina powder to his meat. The smaller the dog is the smaller the pinch should be. You can also purchase dog vitamins from pet shops or the local veterinary surgeon.

This type of plant is found in freshwater and is high in nutrients. Spirulina has a number of nutrients such as vegetable protein, carbohydrates, vitamin A, B complex, D and K.

Be sure to add it to the meat after you have placed the meat in his bowl. Do not add it to the entire weeks supply of meat.

Turmeric Powder Benefits

Turmeric can be a great inflammation reducer used in small doses. Here in Australia you find it in the same place as the powered curry, herbs and spice section of the supermarket.

As Mark Antony got older - his joints would ache, for this reason, I gave him a tinny pinch of Turmeric in his food three times a week.

Note:
If you know your dog has a slow heart beat then do not add lavender.
If your dog has a heart conditions of any kind do not add the essential oil of-Thyme. Replace the Thyme with one extra drop of Eucalyptus.

Epilepsy and Seizures

Ice will be:- both your dog and your own saving grace.
Place an ice pack in the middle of their back.

Treating Dog Seizures & Canine Epilepsy Naturally

If a dog starts having a seizure, or you sense he is about to have one, run to your freezer and grab an ice pack (or in a pinch, a bag of frozen vegetables will work just as well). Hold the ice pack in the middle of his back, and move it back and forth slightly up and down the spinal cord. I've found if you get ice on there within the first 30 seconds of a seizure, it will usually stop almost immediately. Without the ice, the seizure may go on for several minutes. In addition, I've noticed the ice seems to prevent the dog from being in a "fog" after a seizure. A full-length seizure is hard on an animal, and they can be in a daze for hours or even a day or two after. Using an ice pack seems to prevent this. If your dog sleeps far from the freezer at night, consider keeping an ice pack in a small cooler next to your bed, to have ready in an emergency.

When I first started this book, both my dogs were very healthy. Mark Antony last year turned seventeen. This year in February 2017 I found the need to send him to heaven. However, when he first started having his seizures I found it very beneficial to use ice packs on his back. During his first two seizures I was very upset and in shock. After each seizure, he was dazed for over an hour and very confused for the next few days. He appeared to have gone blind. Then a few hours later, he got his sight back. Over the following week his seizures became longer and more frequent. Ice packs did stop the seizures more quickly and he was less dazed. His sight was better than when I had not used the ice packs.

However, he had brain cancer and there was no cure for him at his age. It has taken me a long time to write this section in this book. It is seven months since he left me and it is still very painful to write about.

Some dogs take fits and live a long life when treated with natural products. If your dog takes fits or has epilepsy seek a natural alternative.

Checkout this website.
http://dog.rescueme.org/seizures

Ice packs are amazing. I fell off the roof of my campervan once and landed on my posterior. The back of my head bounced as I hit the ground. I could hear a loud bang as the back of my head bounced on the grass. I came too, crawled to the fridge put lots of ice - on my head, then called the ambulance. The doctors were amazed that there was no swelling on or around my brain. My head was not pounding either. I do have tendinitis now but , at least the ice stopped the main damage.

Bathing Your Dog.

Please do not use the garden hose unless it is summer time and be sure it is only a gentle spray of water. Another point to remember is to test the temperature of the water coming out of the hose. On cool days, the water in the hose could be freezing cold. On warm days, the water that comes out of the hose within the first few minutes may be boiling hot.

Shampoo Types.

My thirteen year old Mark Antony has very sensitive skin. I have tried all kinds of shampoos from the most expensive to the cheapest. There does not appear to be any difference in how his skin reacts so now I purchase the cheapest and add some Essential oils. As soon as I purchase the shampoo I add one drop of Essential oil of Lavender and one drop of Eucalyptus. Shake the bottle well and keep in a dark cool cupboard. Sometimes I use, Oatmeal soap or Olive oil soap from the health food store. If your dog has sensitive skin, see my section headed sensitive skin. Also, when I am in the mood I make shampoo for him. The recipe is below.

Note this book is now revised and its 2017 Mark Antony is seventeen and a half years old.

Bath time should not be a quick let's get this job out of the way scenario. This is the time each week that you get to nurture and explore lots of things about your dog. Sure, there are times when he needs a quick bath or rinse but his weekly bath ritual should be pleasing to him and helpful to you in his long term maintenance plan.

If you bath the dog in your bathtub place a towel on the bottom of the bath. This will prevent him from scratching the bath and stop him from slipping.

Be sure you have everything ready.

1) Bristle brush
2) Rake comb
3) Soft toothbrush
4) Shampoo
5) Eye drops (for dogs with sensitive eyes)
6) Shower hose {attached to tap}
7) Hand towel for the base of the bath
8) Small Face cloth to cover his eyes.
9) Towel for the dog
10) Clean collar and lead

In a bucket of warm water add half a cup of vinegar and 1 drop of essential oil of Eucalyptus mixed with 1 teaspoon of olive oil. Set this aside for the final rinse. Put a mug in the bucket. The mug is used for collecting the water and poring over your dog. Do not put this rinse water on his face.

Now you have everything ready begin the bath.

Brush Your Dogs Coat.

Start brushing your dog with the bristle brushes to sooth him in the same direction as his coat sits. Then comb gently with the rack comb and try to remove knots. Never start the knot removal at the skin. Start at the end of the knot and work your way back to the skin.

Place a towel on the base of the bath.

Place your dog on the towel.

Rinse the dog with warm running water. While you are rinsing your dog, you should check for fleas and flea eggs. As the running water parts his hair also check for other conditions of his skin. This is the time to try to comb or brush the fleas down the drain.

At this point if your dog has sensitive eyes put the eye drops in his eyes. I use one drop in each eye on my dogs Mark Antony and Ceasar of Viscotears you purchase it from the local Chemist. I keep it in the refrigerator for up to three months.

Place some shampoo on a bristle brush.

Brush the dog's body from the neck down to the end of his tail. Then brush his stomach. Next, you brush his Legs, paws and nails.

During this process rinse the brush to remove dirt and fleas and flea eggs from the brush. You will also need to add extra water and shampoo to the brush.

Leave the shampoo on the body and legs, while you do the face neck and ears. Clean his face with a soft toothbrush.

Now rinse his face neck and ears. You need to be careful not to get water inside his ears nor up his nose. I like to put bubs in my dogs ears or hold my thumb in their ears while I rinse.

The water should be cooler for the face and ears. Otherwise, you will burn his eyes and the skin on the ears. I like to point the hose away from his face like they do in a Hairdressing salon. When I do the face I do so with the water pressure lowered and I have a cotton pad over my dogs eyes.

The body brush can be used on the outside of his ears, the top of his head and his neck. But only use a soft toothbrush around the eyes and his mouth. I place my thumb over my dog's eyes while brushing around his eye.

As you gently work your way around his face and ears rinse each section as soon as you have washed it. Be prepared to get splashed your dog will immediately shake the water from his head.

Use the soft toothbrush to remove dirt from his inner ear flap. With your finger press on his ear cavity while you rinse his inner ear flap to prevent water going down inside his ear.

Now use the shower hose to rinse his entire face and ears.

Depending on the size of your dog use either the soft toothbrush or the body brush to shampoo around his neck then his mouth.

Rinse off the shampoo from his neck and mouth. Rinse both brushes. Now as you rinse the entire body brush him as you rinse.

Reach for the towel before you finish rinsing him. Place the towel around your neck. Now turn off the water and use your hands to remove excess water from his coat.

Use the mug to pour the vinegar water over the entire body. I use cotton wool to place some of the vinegar water around his face and ears. At this point you need to be mindful of his eyes. If this mixture seeps into his eyes they will burn for a few days. I try to hold a hand towel over his eyes. Using the cotton wool pads gives you more control of how much vinegar goes onto his face.

Now towel dry your dog and put on his clean collar and lead.

Walk him around for a few minutes as he will want to shake. Give him a treat and tell him what a good dog he is.

Now use a blow dryer to complete the drying process and give him a good brushing down.

When you have completed his grooming be sure to rinse the brushes in very hot water. Now rinse the brush in vinegar then place the brush in the sun to dry. Do the same with the two brushes you used to bath the dog. Vinegar kills lice and fleas.

Now inspect your dogs' teeth and gums. It's important to note the colour each week of your dogs' gums. If your dog should ever become ill his gums will change colour.

If his teeth need cleaning then set some time aside within a few days to clean his teeth. Use a soft toothbrush and the inside flesh of a banana skin. The inside flesh of a banana skin is also a great tooth whitener for you and your family. More on your dogs teeth and gums can be read under the headings "Gums" and "Teeth"

See Daily Health Check.

Nails

A very important part of a dogs grooming is to cut his nails at least once a month, so as to only need to cut the tips off. Some dogs have white nails like us and the quick is very easy to see.

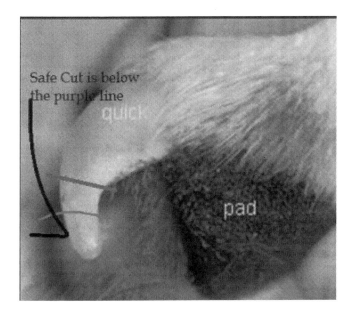

Safe Cut is below the purple line

quick

pad

Other dogs with black nails are very concerning as you cannot see the quick. For this reason It is best to cut just the very tip of the nail and do it often.

Should you cut the quick, put corn starch on the tip. I add one drop of Rose geranium to the corn starch to the corn flower/starch. Borax is what the Vets use but I do not like that to be placed on an open wound.

Then place gauze over the tip and a bandage.
I would then give the dog a pain killer.

Go to Washington Uni website for a full review on cutting dogs nails.

http://www.vetmed.wsu.edu/outreach/Pet-Health-Topics/categories/procedures/dogs/clipping-your-dog's-claws

If you type into Google Washington Pet Uni their site comes up. Then in the top left corner there is a little magnifier symbol. Click that and type in cutting dogs nails.

Bathing a Dog With Sensitive Skin

All the above instructions are the same but the most important issue for dogs with sensitive skin is to massage him with essential oil massage mix before you begin to brush him. The second point is oil does not mix with water that is why you then need to put the soap or shampoo on and massage that in then rinse him.

So lets be clear on this.
- Massage him with the massage oil.
- Bush him
- Put shampoo on and massage in
- Now rinse with warm water.
- Then the vinegar rinse.

Final vinegar rinse is a bucket of warm, not hot water with a tablespoon of vinegar added to it. Never get this in his eyes it will sting and burn his eyes. I use a cup as a dipper and pour this rinse over him one cup at a time. When I do the outside of his ears I put a face cloth firmly over his eyes.

Fleas and other mites do not like vinegar.

Sensitive Skin Pre-Bath Massage Oil.

- In 100 ml of Olive oil add:-
- 1 drops of Eucalyptus Essential oil.
- 3 drops of Chamomile Essential oil
- 3 drops of Rose Geranium Essential oil

Keep this mix in a dark bottle in a cool dark place. Not the refrigerator.

Note : if it is a lovely warm day I massage Mark Antony with this oil mix about half an hour before I bath him and leave him outside to play. This gives the oil mix time to enter through to the deeper layers of his skin.

Just moments before his bath get everything ready, as I have explained above.

Place him in the bath on the towel.

Pour a little of the mix all the way down his back bone and put some in your hands.

Work the oil into his skin.

With a soft hairbrush, brush his entire body.

Dip the brush into the bucket of water and vinegar. As prepared per the above instructions. Only use half the vinegar mix. Add some shampoo to the brush and brush the dog; you may have to dip the brush into the bucket of water several times to get the shampoo to lather. Now continue as above with his bath time ritual.

It is very important to note that hosing the dog while the oil is on his body is a big, "no". Oil does not mix with water. You need to emulsify the oil with the shampoo or soap first.

Brushing Your Dog

Every day you should spend about 10 to 15 minutes brushing your dog and once a week about 40 to 60 minutes. Naturally, it takes less time to brush a dog with short hair than it does to brush a dog with long or curly hair.

There are good reasons to brush your dog daily. It creates bonding between you and stimulates his lymphatic system. It allows you to check for fleas and ticks, removes knots which can tug at their skin. Always start with the bristle brush. Brush in the opposite direction to how the hair / fur lays.

Brushing and combing also helps keep your dog's coat and skin healthy and looking good. Whether you go from tail to head or head to tail is entirely up to you. It is important to remove loose hairs with the rack comb being very careful not to pull through the knots. Be very gentle around the anus under the tail, the tail tip, ears and eyes.

If you do not take the time you will pay the price. The dog could have a nest of fleas biting into his skin which causes skin irritation, the mange and heart worms. He could have a tick and that would be fatal.

Dogs Ears

At the first sign of any rash or skin irritation in your dogs ears apply this mixture.

100 ml Olive oil
add 10 drops essential oil of Rose Geranium.
Gently massage the inside of his ear flap, with a tiny amount of this mix.

To know more about dogs ears read this info:-
https://www.vetmed.wsu.edu/outreach/Pet-Health-Topics/categories/procedures/dogs/examining-and-medicating-the-ears-of-your-dog

Bites

My Dog Was Bitten By?

If you do not know, what, has bitten the dog and you are sure it was not a snake, put some vinegar on the bite. Press the area with some ice wrapped in paper towel. Try to hold it on the area for at least five minutes. Now inspect the bit. If it was a bee there could be a small dark spike in the wound that needs to be removed. You can usually pull it out with your fingers or a pair of tweezers. The good thing about spider or insect bites is the sting and the dog will lick the wound. With a snake bite, there is often no immediate pain.

If it was a bull-ant, or some other ant. The area should now look fine within a few minutes. After the vinegar treatment the dog would appear to be happy. However, check his gums to be sure he is feeling alright. See gums

Occasionally anaphylactic shock could develop in a dog that has been stung in the past. You could try reducing the fever with a cool bath (do not put cold water near his head) and a massage of Eucalyptus and lavender oil. They must be essential oils not fragrant oils.

To one tablespoon of cooking oil or butter add 1 drop of Essential oil of Lavender and one drop of Chamomile. Massage this into his stomach. Give him a cuddle and pat him for at least 20 minutes. Check his gums by pressing your finger on the gum if the colour returns within a heartbeat, he is going to be OK.

Should he still be shaking and feverish take him to the Vet immediately. See gums

Shock Mix

My favorite mix when they have a fever or are in shock is:-

In 100 ml bottle of olive oil or cold pressed grape-seed oil add:-
1 drop of Essential oil of Lavender
6 drop of Chamomile.

Keep this mix in a dark narrow glass bottle.
If your dog has low blood pressure do not use the Lavender oil in the mix.

Pat this mix on the wound and massage his stomach with the rest of the mix. Put a cold cloth on his back and cuddle him. If your dog has low or high blood pressure, replace the Lavender oil with Chamomile.

Spider Bite.

Anti-venom for two of our more dangerous spiders, the funnel-web and the redback has been available since the 1950s and 1981, respectively. It is only administered when the envenomation is severe, which is rarely the case.

Spider venom contains a cocktail of chemicals, some of which can be harmful to humans - but humans are not really the intended victims. Spider venom is designed for small prey and delivered in small quantities that, while often fatal to tiny creatures, can be handled by bigger organisms. When injected to a horse, for instance, spider venom triggers the animal's immune system to produce antibodies to fight the effect of the toxin.

If you are sure it was a spider bite see if you can capture the spider in a jar and put the lid on. The vet may need to see the spider. Most household spiders are not dangerous. Treat the same way as explained above for an ant bit.

If you expect it was a dangerous type of spider you will need to see a vet immediately. If you cannot afford a Vet nor get to one give your dog as much help as you can.

Wash the bite with warm water. Rub his stomach with the above Essential oil mix. Do not put ice on the bite. Repeat this procedure every hour. Give him a quarter of an Aspro. Be sure the Aspro is a buffered Aspro. Cuddle him a lot do not brush or stroke him. See Aspirin/Aspro

Treating a venomous bit and ant or bee sting are treated differently. No ice pack when it is venomous but, ice pack can be used when it is non- venomous.

If You Get Bitten By A Dog.

Immediately wash the wound.

If it is a sallow wound, wash and apply an ice pack. If it is a surface wound apply an antiseptic. I use a teaspoon of olive oil and one drop of eucalyptus oil.

If it is a deep wound you will need Tetanus shot? Wash the wound and apply the above mix or vinegar. Ring your Doctor or go to the local hospital for your tetanus shot.

Snake Bite.

Snake bites are a real risk for pets, particularly families that live in the bush. The severity of the bite is dependent upon the species of snake and whether the snake injected venom or simply performed a 'dry bite' (no venom released). A large percentage of bites are dry and this usually occurs because snakes don't consider humans to be prey and have no intention of eating you. Hence, they want to save their venom if possible. Bites tend to occur more frequently in dogs and usually involve the head, neck, and paws. This is due to the inquisitive and brave nature of dogs.

Signs

You might hear your dog yelp. Ran to him as you would a child. Cuddle him and calm him.

Direct observation of interaction between dog and snake in conjunction with a bite wound or evidence of trauma (limp or bleeding)

- Pain
- Lameness
- Swelling
- Bruising and Bleeding
- Lethargy and Weakness
- Tremors and Seizures
- Vomiting and Diarrhea
- Action Plan

If you suspect a snakebite, try to implement the following:

Ensure you and your family are safe and the snake is no longer in the vicinity.

Calm your pet down as quickly as possible. Muzzle if necessary but ensure collar and muzzle are loose enough that there is no constriction. If any constriction, remove all items immediately.

Immobilize the part of the animal that has been bitten and try to avoid elevating it.

Drive to your nearest vet clinic immediately.

Suggestions

Try to identify the snake without putting you or others at risk. If you are 100% comfortable that the snake is dead, take a photo or Carefully bring the snake in for identification by your Veterinarian. Knowledge of the species is important to ensure the Vet uses the correct anti-venom.

Don't try to kill the snake.

Do not manipulate the affected area of the bite any more than necessary.

Don't let your pet roam around freely.

Don't administer any medication without your vet's consultation.

I have not had this happen to anyone nor any of my animals but if you have eucalyptus oil handy pour a drop on the wound and rush to the vet.

Because snakebites are rear, there is not enough research around. In the olden days they had a pen in the first aid kit. It was a tiny Sharpe knife. Similar, in shape and size to a sewing un-picker. They would cut the wound and make it bleed. The other end of this pen shaped instrument contained a small amount of crushed charcoal to place on the wound. They would first place a strap {a tourniquet} above the wound and tie tight to stop the poison from travelling towards the heart.

If you are nowhere near a vet, you could try this. You could use a razor blade to cut the wound and put one drop of eucalyptus on after you have made the wound bleed. Do not apply a tourniquet as they have found that causes other toxic issues when it, is taken off. Do apply a bandage firmly but not tightly to the bite. Ring a vet and ask what you could do.

Warning
They now say you must not disturb the wound. Old farmers here in Australia would tell you, as I have, to make it bleed.
However, you need to decide, if you are not close to a vet. Read this information.

https://www.ehp.qld.gov.au/wildlife/livingwith/snake s/snake_bites.html

http://www.dogslife.com.au/dog-news/dog-health/what-to-do-if-your-dog-is-bitten-by-a-snake
Signs your dog has been bitten

Dr Sillince says, it may be hard to identify the symptoms of a snake bite because it will all depend on the type of snake that has bitten your dog.

"The animal will probably start shaking and madly vomiting or start bleeding, depending on what it has been bitten by," says Dr Sillince. "You will know it's an emergency and you'll suspect it's a snake bite. It's a much quicker process than ticks."

Symptoms of a venomous snake bite are very much like the symptoms of a paralysis tick.
According to the Australian Veterinary Association (AVA), symptoms include:-

- Sudden weakness followed by collapse
- Bleeding puncture wound
- Swelling in the bitten area
- Pain and discomfort
- Neurological signs such as twitching, drooling and shaking
- Vomiting

- Loss of bladder and bowel control
- Dilated pupils
- Paralysis

If you see the above signs, or suspect your dog may have been bitten by a snake, make sure to keep your pooch calm and take it to the vet immediately.

Treating The Snake Bite

"The first aid rules on snake bites have changed. They have changed for humans as well, but they've changed differently for dogs. The rule for dogs is just get in the car and drive," says Dr Sillince.

She says there are a couple of reasons for this:

1. You do not know where the dog has been bitten and you can waste 15 minutes trying to find the bite, which is time that could have been spent getting the dog to the vet.
2. If the dog dies on the way to the vet, it was going to die anyway. In other words, it was already too late.
3. Dogs have fur, which makes pressure bandaging very difficult because the fur acts as a buffer and stops the bandage from properly tightening.
4. There are some slight differences in the way the lymphatics work in dogs, versus humans.

In humans, when you pressure bandage, you are essentially stopping the lymphatic system, but there is less evidence of that working in dogs.

"So, the only rule for snake bites in dogs is: if you are within 20 minutes to half an hour of a veterinary surgery, keep the animal calm, keep yourself calm and get in the car and drive. Ring the vet and let them know you're coming. Make sure to have your vet on speed dial – this is very handy in emergencies," says Dr Sillince.

If you are travelling with your dog know where a vet is in that area. Googleing the info takes precious time. Read these articles before your dog gets bitten and have some of these items in your first aid kit.

http://www.barkingbotanicals.com.au/dog-bitten-snake/

"Do not do the 'typical' owner thing of 'oh, the vet costs a lot of money, we'll just wait until tomorrow and see how it goes.' You'll likely lose the dog or multiply the bill by 10. If the animal is wheezing, it's alertness response or its brightness response is down, move like 'Greased Lightning'. The vet bill will be less if you move quickly."

The majority of snake bite cases end with the animal surviving, which is why it is so important to get your dog to the vet immediately.

"The recovery rate from snake bites is pretty good," explains Dr Sillince. "There is some pretty sophisticated veterinary technology nowadays and the antivenins are sound. They're very available. There is a little bit of a risk with antivenins but really not a lot. They are very high quality. So it's a case of being alert but not alarmed."

How To Avoid A Snake

Most times when I am walking in bushland or paddocks with long grass I make a lot of noise and have a small tree branch that I shuffle along the ground in front of me.

Most of the time, snakes will likely want to avoid you, especially if you have your dog with you. Snakes don't like being around dogs, as they are seen as predators, so they won't voluntarily go into areas where there are dogs. For example, if you've got a yard on the edge of the bush and your dogs are in the yard, snakes will rarely go deliberately into the area.

"Snakes think dogs are predators. Most snake attacks happen when the dog is being nosy in a place where it shouldn't or when a dog stands on a snake or gets close enough to frighten the snake into attacking a leg," explains Dr Sillince. "The only real exception is a tiger snake that will go after prey, but tiger snake venom is nothing too drastic and is treatable. The real scary ones are the brown snakes and, further north, the Taipans and Adders."

To reduce the likelihood of coming across a snake, making sure your yard is clean and free of rock or wood piles as well as keeping an eye out if walking through a bushy area, especially in the warmer months.

"Rule one for reducing or avoiding snake bites is to keep your yard clean. In other words, don't have piles of rocks for snakes to set up house in and if you do have a wood pile, fence it off from the dog. You can even get snakes in suburban backyards if you've got piles of rocks or wood,"

"Secondly, if you are walking your dog at dawn or dusk, keep your eyes open. Most snakes are really, visible. I have done plenty of bushwalking and have seen a snake in the middle of the path because it's clear. It's a good spot for a snake to lie, so you just need to keep your eyes open. If your dog is off the lead call him and put him on his lead. Throw a small branch or a stone towards the snake.

"Thirdly, trust your dog. Dogs do recognize snakes as animals and dogs do recognize their tracks. But if you are walking along the path and your dog is in front of you, your dog will generally look in the direction of the snake if it has seen it.

"Lastly, if you have to go into a heavily wooded area and you don't have any other choice, make noise. Stamp your feet because snakes can feel vibrations and they do hear noise, plus they don't like humans. Most snakes will very happily move away."

What To Do If Your Dog Is Attacking A Snake

If you see your dog attacking a snake, don't get involved because you will likely get bitten yourself.

"The first thing I'd do is get a photo if I can because if the dog is fighting a snake, it has probably been bitten and it's the only chance I'll get to identify the snake," she advises. "Now, if you don't know your snakes by eye, you can scream at your dog, throw something at them, anything to get the dog to back away but, I tell you what, if your dog is having a fight with a snake, it is probably pretty serious. Throwing a rock will probably not get the dog to back off. Just make sure to not get involved because you don't want to get bitten by the dog or the snake. You are of no use if you are injured. When the fight settles down, and it's normally pretty quick (around five or 10 seconds of total chaos followed by deathly silence), I would consider taking the dog in the car and getting it checked out by the vet."

Identifying Snakes

Most of the time, the vet will ask whether you were able to spot the type of snake your dog was bitten by. However, if you didn't see the snake, or don't know what type it was, don't panic.

"The vets will always ask because they must but in the vast majority of cases, the owner does not know. And in the vast majority of cases, the antivenin that's used, if it's used, is multivalent antivenin, unless there's a good reason [not to]."

"The further north you go, the more likely it is that you'll see taipans and adders. In coastal zones, you're more likely to get whip snakes or brown or black snakes, and in the agricultural belt, you're more likely to see brown snakes, so vets can take an educated guess to know what type of snake it is by the reports they are getting.

"But, most often, they will use a multivalent antivenin or in an increasing number of cases now, they will simply treat the symptoms. If it's a poisonous snake, it will produce symptoms that is the definition of poison. If it is a non-poisonous snake, let's say a very, very low-venomous snake, such as a little whip snake, you'll get local swelling, pain and distress, but you won't get any of those horrible symptomatic neurotoxicities that you will from the more poisonous snakes."

Car Accidents

When your darling pet, is hit by a moving vehicle this usually means a rush to the Veterinary clinic. There are many different situations when your dog, is hit by a moving vehicle. The speed and type of vehicle make an enormous difference to the severity of the situation.

A car that has had the suspension lowered may hit your dog with the bumper and send your dog flying. Depending on how the dog lands and his weight, this may not cause too much damage depending on the size of the dog.

A car with flat tyres may run over the dog and will not cause as much damage as a car with fully inflated tyres. A bus or truck may run over the top of the dog without too much damage at all providing the dog has been in the middle of the vehicle. Your dog will have an adrenalin rush and run to you or the side of the road. This does not mean the dog is all right. This is what they do if they do not have any major broken bones. However, even if they have major brakes in their bones, some dogs are still able to run to safety and then they flop.

If your dog is in a critical state it will not be able to move from the position it landed after the accident. Oh boy oh boy I hate to talk about this but if the dog is critical you will need to drive him to the vet to be put to sleep and allow him to leave you and go to his maker.

If you are completely broke and unable to get the assistance of your vet do this. On some occasions, you may be able to nurse the dog back to good health yourself. Naturally, if you can afford to it is best to have the veterinary check your dog over.

If the dog has a noticeable area that is swollen put ice on that area. Hold the dog in a way he feels safe and happy and keep the ice on for several minutes. Talk to him in a gentle manner and stroke him. Holding an ice pack on his back should also calm him.

Once he is calm check his gums. Press the gum above the front teeth. The gum should go whitish under your finger and as you release a second later his gum should turn back to its normal colour instantly. If it is slow to return the dog is in trauma.

Apply one tablespoon of olive oil with 2 drops of Chamomile essential oil to his stomach and a cold wet cloth to his head. Bath any wound with a mix of warm water and a pinch of salt. It is important not to let him fall to sleep while you are nurturing him. Keep cuddling him and talking to him for about ten minutes.

1. **Take his pulse. See dogs pulse**

2. **Smell his breath.**

You now need to check his gums again. If the blood returns quickly you can now check to see if he has any broken bones or sprains. Gently work your way over his entire body pressing and moving his legs. If he yelps very loudly check that spot again to work out if it is a sprain or a break. If the dog has a sprain put ice on that section. If you think it is a break he needs urgent attention.

Check the dogs pulse. See **Dogs pulse**

Have a smell of their breath if it is worst than normal they are probable bleeding internally. Dogs do have bad breath most of the time even if you give them bones and clean their teeth on a regular basis. That is why I check their breath each day.

There are some veterinary surgeons, that will fix your dog for a reduced fee and they will allow you to make small weekly payments. If these payments would cause you great hardship then you would be best to have your dog put to sleep or surrender him to the RSPCA.

I know that is tough love but right at this moment it is about the dogs not you. The love you have for him and the amount of joy he has given you means you have to do what is best for him not what is best for you.

Ceasar Was Hit By A Car

Ceasar was hit by a car, in a free rest stop while we were travelling around Australia. We had just got out of the campervan to stretch our legs. The young driver came in off the highway racing around the area like a speedway driver. The driver almost hit me as I was putting the lead on Ceasar. Ceasar went flying into the air. He yelped /screamed like he was a child that had been hit. He came running back to me and fell down at my feet.

There was no ice in my camp refrigerator. We were three hundred kilometers from a vet. My mobile phone, was out of range and I was beside myself.

His mouth was bleeding and he had lost a tooth. I quickly picked Ceasar up and placed a cold piece of steak that was in a plastic bag on his back and massaged him with my essential oil of Chamomile. Chamomile is purchased in 10 ml bottles it is 3% Chamomile in Jojoba oil and safe to apply without mixing as it is already mixed with base oil. I checked his gums and smelt his breath. His breath was normal.

If they have a very bad smell to their breath worst than normal it indicates they are bleeding internally. After about ten minutes he had stopped shaking so I checked to see if anything was broken. This is one good reason to keep your dogs teeth clean.

I checked his pulse it was a little faster than normal.

I then drove until my mobile had range and I searched the internet for a vet. Thank the heaven above, for smart phones anyone that does not have one should get one.

It was 6 pm by this time and the vet had a message service. I left a message and he rang me back about ten minutes later. The vet slowly went through all the vital signs with me and it seemed that Ceasar was doing fine. I made an appointment to have the vet check Ceasar out the next morning. I then drove to the next rest stop where there were other gray nomads camping for the night.

There I checked Ceasar over again. He was happy to come for a walk and eat some of his dinner. He also showed signs of being interested in other dogs that were there with the campers. However, I did not allow him to play with them.

One lovely couple could see I was stressed and offered for me to have dinner with them. That was a blessing because I was in no state to cook for myself and could not eat much.

The next morning I left early and drove another 200 kilometers to have the vet look at Ceasar. Amazingly, all Ceasar needed was some pain relief. That was two and a half years ago and we are all doing fine. Ceasar, amazingly, was reasonably unharmed.

Chicken Casserole

In a large pot put:-

- One medium size chicken
- 1 carrot
- 1 stick of celery
- 1 tiny knob of garlic see note below.
- Some green leafy vegetables
- A small piece of pumpkin
- 2 large potatoes
- 1 cup of peas
- A small brunch of parsley
- Add a few fresh mint leaves after cooking.

Cover with water and bring to the boil. Now reduce heat, then simmer for another twenty minutes with the lid on the saucepan. See below for further instructions.

Add some chopped mint after you have finished cooking.

Garlic is actually a poison for dogs so only use this if your dog has a very serious disease. Only give this casserole for a few days. Then make a new batch without the garlic.

For a large dog you can double or triple the ingredients. If he is slightly unwell then you could add some boiled rice to his dish with the casserole. But, do not add rice if he needs a few day to get his energy back or is convalescing after an operation.

Never add rice to the soup nor his casseroles. Rice goes off within a day or two, and will send the soup or casserole off. It is best to cook rice separately and store separately - then add as required.

Cover the ingredients with water. Bring to the boil then lower the heat put the lid on the pot and simmer for one and a half hours.

Remove the chicken, place on a chopping board and remove all the bones. Break all the chicken into tiny pierces. Set aside with a cloth over the top.

Drain off some of the broth from the pan and put into a 24 ice block tray. Put into your freezer.

Mash the vegetables in the pan with the rest of the broth.

Add the boned chicken pierces to the pan add another cup or two of water and bring to the boil. Stir in a little rice powder to thicken. Do not add the rice powder for very sick dogs that you have to feed with a pipette.

Add the chopped mint.

Put half this chicken casserole into the freezer and half into the refrigerator. When you have just one meal left in the refrigerator, take the rest out of the freezer.

Give the dog a small amount of the chicken casserole each morning and a larger quantity each night. Give him a chicken broth ice block every few hours.

The ice blocks help to keep his temperature down.

Chicken Broth For A Sick Dog

If your dog is refusing to eat because he is very ill do this:-

First understand that this casserole/stew/broth is only for animals that have contracted a disease and can only be given for three days. After the third day give him normal chicken broth see recipe below. The Garlic will fight the disease but will also make him vomit.

When you remove the chicken, also remove the vegetables.

Make the ice blocks with the broth. For big dogs put some broth into plastic zip bags, and stand them in a square plastic container and freeze. You may need to cut the bag open if the larger ice blocks do not come out of the bag. With the remaining broth, try to get him to have some every hour.

You may have to buy a pipette and gently squirt some of the broth onto his tongue every hour. You may also have to break up the ice block and put small amount onto his tongue every 10 minutes or so. When you go to bed at night give him some more broth and Aspirin/Aspro. Then give him some chicken broth to which you have added a pinch (1/8 teaspoon) of electrolyte powder.

Leave a chicken ice block on a small dish with some of the broth close to his bed. In another bowl put water with 1/8 teaspoon of electrolyte powder. Be sure to set your alarm and get up every four hours to administer the broth. Remember as I have stated above only give him the soup for a few days with garlic. Garlic is a poison to dogs.

This mix I gave to Ceasar, when he was just 3 months old. He was attacked by two large dogs just a week before his second injection. He seemed find just a few cuts and in his skin and shaken-up by the experience but a few days he did a green waterish bowel motion (poo) and collapsed. He had contracted Parvo. After two Vets telling me he had to be put down this broth I used to save his life. There are times when garlic needs to be given but, it is not something you should use all the time.

 If your dog is very dehydrated, you will need to give him the broth and an electrolyte every hour or take him to a veterinary to have a drip put in. See heading "Dehydrated dog."

Should you need a nurse for eight to ten hours a day and your family are all busy hire a granny. You can advertise on www.gumtree.com.au for a local retired person, ask a neighbor, and put a sign up in your local pet shop and on a nearby bus stop shed.

Dogs Need Grandparents.

Do not wait till your dog gets sick to organize a granny to help with your dogs care. Would you leave a sick child with a complete stranger? I have four lifelines for my dogs.

My daughter if I need to go somewhere on the weekends. A retired lady if my daughter is not going to be home. This lady only charges me twenty dollars to take care of my dogs over night. A dog walker who will come twice a day. The cost is just twenty five dollars. When my mum was alive she helped with several of my sick dogs over many decades.

It is important that there is an envelope with some money in it hidden in your home. If the dog gets sick while you are away the dog walker or the retired career may need to get the dog to a Vet. If they do not want to use their car or they do not have a car they will need taxi money. In this day and age, you can use your visa card to pay the Vet over the telephone or the Vet can send a PayPal invoice to your smart phone. However, you could book the taxi and pay over the telephone. Then these life lines will be in place should your dog need care while you are at work.

Electrolytes For Dogs

A dog may need electrolyte replacement when he's dehydrated from diarrhea or blood loss. A wound that bleeds heavily is a true emergency, while bloodsuckers on the outside, such as fleas and ticks, or on the inside, such as hookworms and tapeworms, are a long-term problem that can precipitate an equally urgent crisis. Either way, the dog needs immediate help to restore the content and balance of sodium and chloride in his bloodstream.

Dogs Don't Always Need Electrolytes.

A dog doesn't need electrolyte replacement when he's been exercising, even exercising very hard. When humans sweat to cool themselves, they lose salt (sodium chloride) and other minerals in their sweat. Since dogs don't sweat through their skin, they cool themselves by panting, which evaporates only water from their tongues. They don't lose any minerals this way and need only water replacement, without the electrolytes.

Store-Bought Versus Homemade Electrolytes

Commercial electrolyte-balancing solutions for dogs are readily available through veterinarians and even on the Internet, but these may contain things a dog doesn't really need, mainly preservatives to keep them shelf-stable. With homemade electrolyte water, he can get the essential ingredients without anything he might be sensitive to.

Make Your Own Electrolyte.

Electrolyte water needs to be made in careful proportions so as not to give a dog too much of anything. Sodium and chloride are already in correct proportion in ordinary table salt, so one teaspoonful of table salt dissolved in a quart of clean, fresh water will create an electrolyte replacement appropriate for a dehydrated dog. This mixture contains all he really needs in an emergency, but adding a tablespoonful of sugar or honey may make it more palatable to him without doing any harm. You can open a can of good-quality low-sodium chicken broth and dilute it with two cans of water; this lowers the sodium content enough that it will not hurt the dog and he may be more willing to take it with this flavoring.

Chicken Stock

The ultimate restorative for a sick or injured dog is homemade chicken stock made with chicken necks, backs and wingtips simmered slowly for eight hours or until the bones crumble, then strained and seasoned with kitchen herbs (parsley, sage, thyme and the like, but no onion or garlic) and a measured teaspoon of salt per quart. This has actual easily digested protein content and is attractive to dogs in smell and taste. After you steam for an hour put through a clean cloth so there is only the liquid remaining.

Common Dog Dangers

Prevention Is Key When Trying To Keep Your Dog Safe From Everyday Dangers: Keep him where you can control what he does. Do not wait for him to become ill before you act. Take care of him daily as you would a child.

Coughing And Causes

Allergic Reaction To Food.

It could be he is allergic to his food and that causes the throat to swell and he starts coughing. If this is correct he will always cough about 10 to 20 minutes after he eats then the coughing will stop soon after. He may also get a fit of sneezing. This is a clear sign he is allergic to the food you are giving him.

Kennel Cough

Give him a teaspoon of Honey he will love it. I usually crush up quarter of a baby Aspirin and add to the honey. Make him some chicken soup see the recipe under my heading Chicken Casserole. Give him only the chicken soup morning and night for a three days then the Chicken Stock until he starts to recover.

Steam Inhalation.

This can be done two ways.

Put a liter of boiling water in a bucket add 6 drops of eucalyptus or a tablespoon of Vicks Vapor rub in the boiling water. Get a blanket, you and your dog get under the blanket with his face close to the bucket. Try to stay under there with him for at least three minutes, six minutes is better.

Or

Put him into the bathroom with the hot water running in the shower. Put some Eucalyptus oil in an oil burner. Sit the burner somewhere safe. Close the door and leave him in the steaming bathroom for 10-20 minutes. You may have to sit in there with him.

Hot water in the bath within 3 drops of Eucalyptus oil will also create healing vapors.

Rub his throat 3 times a day with a mix made up of one tablespoon of olive oil and 1 drop of Eucalyptus oil.

Under my sink I store a 750 gram bottle of Olive oil to which I have added

- 1 drop of Eucalyptus oil
- 1 drop of Lavender
- 1 drop of Peppermint Essential oil.

It has a tag with the amount of Essential oils added and the date I made it on the tag. This mix can be used for you and your dog. It is a great mix to apply to your stomach and the dogs once a week. All you need is a quarter of a teaspoon in the palm of your hand rub your palms together and massage into the stomach. You can store this mix for up to two years in a dark cool cupboard.

If he cuts himself put a pinch of salt in a dish of warm water and bath the cut. I use a clean makeup sponge dip it into the salty water and squeeze over the cut or abrasion several times. Pat dry with tissue then apply Eucalyptus oil with a wet cotton pad that I put one drop of the eucalyptus oil onto. You could also simply add one drop of eucalyptus oil to the salty water.

If the cut is deep, you will need to decide for yourself if it needs stitches. If it does then it's off to the vet.

If it's a small deep cut you might be able to take care of it yourself. Shave around the cut. Wash in warm salty water and dry by patting with tissues. Apply pressure to the wound for a few minutes.

If the bleeding stops use some Steri-Strip bandages and pull the cut together. They will not stick to hair or fur so you will need to shave around the wound. You need to pinch the wound together then apply the Steri-Strips.

Daily Health Check

You may think I do not have time for this but it only takes a few minutes and will be the most valuable tool you have ever had it the dog does get sick you will know what is normal for your dog. This could be life saving.

- Check the colour of his gums and his general health. See heading **"Gums"**
- Check his poo morning and night. See heading "Hard Poo"
- Check his pulse.
- Check the amount of urine and the colour.
- Check how he walks and runs.
- Check the height of his two water bowls.
- Check that his interested in his food.
- Brush or comb him and chick for fleas and ticks.

Desexing Benefits For Your Dog

Most dogs that have not been desexed have to cope with sexual frustration and many other problems. A dog is more likely to have a long and healthy life, if desexed. However, I did not get Mark Antony desexed until this year. I needed to reduce the risk of cancer or other diseases of the reproductive organs, such as testicular cancer and prostate diseases in males, and ovarian cysts and tumors, acute uterine infections. Ceasar on the other hand prefers to keep me, in his sight he has never adventured too far. I will probably have him desexed in a year or so.

Desexed dogs tend to be less aggressive, less distressed when confined to a yard and less likely to roam, reducing risks of death or injury on roads or in a dog fight.

Desexing is not the cause of an overweight dog. Not enough exercise and too much food and are the cause.

The costs of desexing are offset by the discounts given on council registration fees for desexed dogs, and less roaming and aggression help prevent impound fees and vet bills. It's also cheaper to desex dogs than to breed dogs – just ask any responsible registered breeder.

Desexing dogs prior to being sold also prevents dogs being acquired for unscrupulous puppy farming. Most City Councils offer desexing subsidies. Discounted desexing is also offered to concession card holders through the

National Desexing Network
Australia Ph 1300 368 992

Other people that help with the cost of desexing are the Animal Welfare League and RSPCA. They do not pay the full amount but they give assistance. If you live in Queensland it will only cost you about eighty dollars at the Animal Hospital. They are near the Dog Pound. Shelter Rd, Coombabah. Telephone 07 5509 9000.

In most Countries you can receive help with getting your dog desexed or help with care and Veterinary bills. In a few Countries they have witch doctors still to this very day. They are white witches of cause.

No matter what Country you live in there is always help at hand just reach out and ask for it.

Mark Antony is a very over sexed dog. One-day mum and I were down the beach in the dog free area. Mark Antony was born on a boat in Broadwater, near Southport in Queensland. So he smells the ocean and gets very excited and he loves to go swimming with us. As mum and I were leaving the water we called him but he was nowhere in sight. We had our shower got dressed and he still was not back. This was very unusual. He would often run along the beach with other dogs but would return when called.

I had my campervan parked near the shower block and thought maybe his under the van. No he wasn't. Mum and I both went in opposite directions to look for him. He was nowhere to be found. I made mum some dinner and a cup of tea and he still had not returned.

Mum and I watched a movie and suddenly there he was. He jumped into the van sat in the driver seat and jumped out of the van again.

I called him he came to me and so did his girl friend. He had picked up a female on heat and invited her home. The pretty Jack Russell had no collar. It was 10 pm Saturday night so we took his girl friend home with us.

On Monday afternoon when I finished work, we went to the Vet to see if she had a microchip. She did so the Vet called the owner and we were able to return her to her very anxious owners. A few months later she had three adorable little puppies.

Mark Antony adventure did turn out alright but, it could have turned out very badly for both the dogs. We were at Ettalong Beach near the Wharf swimming, and the female dog lived three kilometers away. They had both crossed two main roads and several busy streets. When I tried to work out, how Mark Antony had got to the home of the female dog in the first place the female dog owner was unsure. I asked had they been down the beach and she said, no.

She said, my dog just suddenly appeared in her yard and the two dogs suddenly disappeared again. There have been a few times that, Mark Antony has disappeared. One time he was gone for two days and arrived back at 5 am with a female companion. You are probably are wondering why I had not had him desexed sooner. Well, my daughter has a female Maltese and Mark Antony is her mate. If you are not a license breeder, you can save yourself some big headaches and have your dog desexed.

Diarrhea

Immediately rum his tummy with 1 tablespoon of cooking oil and 1 drop of Essential oil of Peppermint and 1 drop of Eucalyptus oil. Be sure not to give him any food for 24 hours. Give him half a Hydrolyte Electrolyte ice block. Within the next twelve hours rub his tummy again with the above oil mix. If he will not eat the Hydrolyte Electrolyte ice block give him some of the chicken broth ice blocks you have in the freezer. See Chicken Casserole

Diarrhea can be caused by a change in food, dirty water or more serious problems. If it is caused by a change in food or something he ate while out walking the above mix will fix the problem.

In conjunction with diarrhea if your dog has any of the following symptoms please seek immediate veterinary advice.

- Fever
- Pain
- Vomiting
- Blood in the diarrhea
- Lethargy or depression
- Weight Loss
- Dehydration
- Loss of appetite
- Foul smelling diarrhea
- Any other sign of illness

If it is Sunday night and you cannot afford the afterhours Vet fees follow the above instructions. But, rub him with the Essential oil mix every three hours and give him quarter of a baby Aspro every six hours followed with half a Hydrolyte Electrolyte Ice Block. If your dog is over 50 Kilos give him a full Aspro and a full Hydrolyte Electrolyte Ice Block.

Read the section on how I cured Ceasar when he contracted the deadly Parvovirus, an terrible disease.

Dehydrated Dog.

You can easily work out if your dog is dehydrated. An ill dog is at high danger of dehydration, since the illness can cause dog diarrhea, dog vomiting, fever and a lack of desire to eat and drink. Dehydration may occur due to an excessive loss of body fluids, is a common and dangerous condition that needs to be immediately addressed. If left untreated, dehydration can lead to serious consequences, including organ failure and death. For this reason, pet parents should learn to recognize the signs of dehydration and how to respond to it with proper dog first aid and veterinary attention. Along with a loss of water, dehydration also typically involves a loss of electrolytes – minerals such a sodium, chloride and potassium.

Since untreated dehydration can lead to organ failure and death, seek immediate medical attention if dehydration is suspected. Depending on the severity, your vet may suggest water with electrolyte products. In extreme cases, intravenous fluids will be administered to replenish your dog's fluids.

Overheating

Heat-related canine conditions can also become life-threatening without immediate treatment. Overheated dogs can suffer heat exhaustion, heat stroke or sudden death from cardiac arrhythmias.

Panting, followed by disorientation and fast, noisy breathing could signal overheating. Other possible signs: Collapsing or convulsing, bright red or blue gums, vomiting and diarrhea. Since field dogs are unlikely to stop hunting or retrieving when they become dangerously hot, owners should watch their dog closely for overheating signs.

If you suspect your field dog or other dogs are overheated, wet him with cool tap water before heading to the veterinarian. Let the office know you're on the way, so a team can be prepared to act quickly.

Your vet may apply alcohol to the ears, foot pads and groin to safely lower the temperature, as well as administer cool IV fluids. For serious overheating, your dog may need a breathing tube and artificial ventilation. Depending on the severity of symptoms, correcting electrolyte imbalances and controlling seizures may also be needed. If organ damage is suspected, hospitalization may be required.

Prevention

Simple precautions can ward off dehydration and overheating. I use chicken or beef ice blocks to help keep my dogs cooler in summer. When you make yourself or your dogs a casserole, add some extra water. When the casserole is almost cooked drain of the excess fluid and put into containers. Place them in the freezer to set. Be sure there has been no onions nor garlic added to the casserole. They can be added to your family casserole, after you have made your dogs ice blocks.

Offer field dogs water at least hourly. Many dogs enjoy hunting so much they run until they collapse. Wobbliness, weakness or collapse are all signs to provide shade and offer small amounts of water. If your dog doesn't improve, seek immediate veterinary attention.

Help your dog beat the heat by encouraging resting and drinking at his leisure. For field dogs, deep, fast-moving lakes, ponds and rivers may be available to provide fresh, cool water. Allow your dog to submerge his body to siphon off the building heat.

Natural Alternatives to Electrolytes

Coconut water is a natural alternative to electrolyte powders. Coconut water comes from the green un-ripened coconut where as coconut milk comes from the ripened coconut. It's the coconut water you will need for dehydrated dogs and people alike can benefit.

Homemade orange juice is another good natural electrolyte but for children and animals that are dehydrated and unwell, you would need to add it to their chicken broth.

Home Make Electrolytes

Other than coconut water and orange juice you can make electrolytes by following the recipe below. However, my children, grandchildren and my dogs will never drink these type of electrolytes. I would always juice an orange, add a pinch of salt, pinch bicarbonate of soda and a pinch of sugar.

Sugar Option

2 quarts /950 ml of water
3-6 teaspoon of sugar
½ teaspoon of salt
½ teaspoon of baking soda
½ teaspoon of salt substitute (potassium salt)

Store in an air tight container for up to 2 days in the refrigerator and use a pipette to administer 5 ml to your dog ever hour for two days.

For humans you can add 1 pack of sugar-free drink flavoring or lemonade.

Sugar-Free Versions

Sugar free: Although adding sugar to your drink will help you keep your energy levels up, it's not a good option for everyone. People on a low-carb diet or people with diabetes, can choose a recipe that doesn't add sugar to the electrolyte drink:

1 quart /950 ml of water

250 ml of orange juice (citrus juice is a natural source of potassium ions)

3 tablespoons of lemon juice

2 sticks of celery juiced

1 apple finely chopped then juiced

¾ teaspoon of salt

Dehydration In Dogs Is Typically Caused By:

- Vomiting
- Diarrhea
- Fever
- Not enough intake of food or water
- Overexposure to heat

Signs of Dehydration in Dogs Include:

- Lack of skin elasticity
- Dry, sticky gums
- Sunken eyes
- Too much or too little urination
- Lethargy

- Slow capillary refill

Delay in capillary refill (the time it takes for your dog's gum to return to its normal colour after you press your finger firmly against it)

How to Determine Dehydration in Dogs

Naturally it is less accurate than a testing from your veterinarian, but a quick at-home physical examination to test the elasticity of your dog's skin can help tell you if your dog is dehydrated.

To Check Dehydration

Do the following:

Gently pull up on the skin at the back of your dog's neck. If the skin does not immediately spring back to its normal position (within 1 or 2 seconds), your dog is dehydrated and needs immediate attention. The longer it takes for the skin to return to its normal position, the more severe the dehydration.

If your dog is older it will be more difficult to accurately perform this test, since older dogs naturally lose some of their skin elasticity. Be aware that accurately determining dehydration in dogs via the skin test is also difficult in overly skinny (malnourished) or obese dogs.

Bear in mind that even if your pet's skin snaps back to normal immediately, he may still be dehydrated. This is because even pets that are dehydrated will have skin that immediately snaps back to normal if the pet is less than 5 percent dehydrated. The higher the level of dehydration, the more pronounced will be the symptoms.

What You Should Do For Dehydration In Dogs

Dehydration in dogs is serious and if left untreated can be fatal. If you suspect that your dog is dehydrated, act quickly.

Your veterinarian will determine the level of your dog's dehydration and the volume of fluids needed to re-hydrate him. Fluids will then most likely be administered either subcutaneously (under the skin) or intravenously for greatest efficiency.

Your veterinarian will typically also ask you questions about your dog's recent eating and drinking habits and physical symptoms, as well as perform.

If you suspect that your dog is dehydrated, be safe and take him to your veterinarian.

However, if he is not vomiting, you could also try giving him Pedialyte, an electrolyte-replacement drink made for infants, which is also safe for dogs.

To avoid dehydration, always make sure that your dog has plenty of clean, fresh water available and that he eats and drinks normally.

If your dog is ill or injured, monitor him closely to make sure he is drinking enough water to replenish fluids lost due to vomiting, diarrhea or fever. Also, be aware that excess fluids are lost as a result of excessive panting or severe drooling. In cases of drooling, the dog's gums may feel moist, even though he is dehydrated.

Dogs Pulse

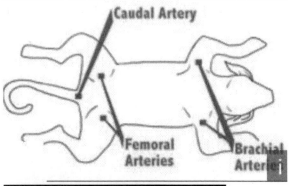

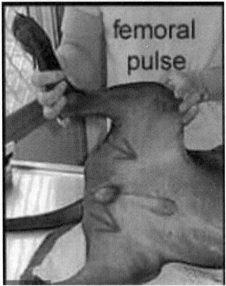

You can feel the femoral artery pumping each time the heart beats.

When you have found the artery with your dog standing, try it with your dog lying on his side. Count how many pulses you feel in 15 seconds and multiply by 4 to get the number of beats per minute.
Dogs normally have a pulse between 70 and 160 beats per minute.

Become familiar with your dog's pulse rate, and how his pulse feels when he is relaxed as well as after exercise.

If you have reason to believe your dog is suffering from an emergency, a dramatic change in pulse (such as, a slowed pulse can indicate shock)

The smaller the dog, the faster its pulse will be. If you believe your dog is in pain, or is ill, and their pulse rate varies significantly from the chart below, take your pet to a veterinarian for medical assistance.

Take the pulse at least two or three times over the next hour. The first few times your pet may get excited or upset at the unfamiliar handling and that would change a normal pulse. Do not wait an hour if it is an emergency. Get them to the vet ASAP.

Allow at least a 5 to 10 beat variance due to generality of sizing chart obesity and age of pet are both factors in gauging answer

Dogs Pulse Ranges

Puppies, the pulse ranges from 120 to 160 beats per minute.

Small Dog - from 140 to 160 beats per minute

Medium Dog - from 120 to 140 beats per minute

Large Dog - from 60 to 80 beats per minute

Dry Skin

There are varying degrees of dry skin. It is hard to use ointments and oils on their skin if they are a house-dog, as the oil will get all over the fabrics and carpets in your home. If you have the time make the below mix and rub into their skin every morning when the sun is out. Leave them out doors until it has settled into their skin. Give them a bone to chew on to occupy their mind. It takes about half a hour for the hair and skin to fully absorb the oil treatment. Then put a cotton or silk dogs coat on them until they have their next bath.

It is important to brush their hair well before you apply the treatment. For dogs with fluffy or long hair part their hair and apply the oil in the parts. Use sparingly a little goes a long way.

Essential oils for dry skin, encourage cellular turnover and stimulate the growth of new cells.

They will gently break down adhesions between skin cells, encouraging the removal of dead skin cells, repairing and healing dull, flaky patches; making them the perfect ingredient for a parched, dry skin. Essential oils for dry skin suit both humans and animals alike.

Properties of Essential Oils

Often a dry skin, is associated with a sensitive skin conditions, such as Eczema, Psoriasis and Dermatitis. Some Essential Oils help to soothe an irritated inflamed skin.

German Chamomile has really wonderful anti-inflammatory properties; others include Lavender, Yarrow, Neroli and my favorites are Rose Otto Rose Geranium and geranium. I have witnessed almost instant skin healings in both humans and animals with Rose Geranium.

Essential Oils for Dry Skin

This is the type of skin that doesn't naturally produce enough sebum (oil).

It can often feel tight and may also be associated with fine lines that run horizontally across the skin. Fortunately there are a number of Essential oils that can help to stimulate the production of sebum, and also balance secretions within the skin.

- Chamomile
- Geranium
- Lavender
- Palma Rosa
- Neroli
- Rose Otto
- Rose Geranium
- Rosewood
- Sandalwood

Oils That Stimulate Circulation

Our skin naturally regulates our body temperature, this it does through a process known as vasodilatations and vasoconstriction, through the superficial capillaries and sudiforous glands.

These glands help to control the production of sweat, whilst regulating body temperature through the evaporation of perspiration. However, dogs do not sweat therefore for human skin you need to follow my recipes in my other books. In this book follow my recipes for carefully and do not change the mixture without the aid of an Aromatherapist.

Essential Oils for dry skin, also play a role in encouraging micro stimulation, within our skin's tissues:

- German Chamomile
- Geranium
- Rose Otto
- Rosemary
- Lemon

Dry Skin Treatment

In 100 ml Olive Oil
Add
5 Drops Rose Geranium.
5 Drops Chamomile

Keep in a cool dark place. Shelf life 2 years.
Note: Because Chamomile is very expensive, it is sold in a mixture of Jojoba oil. The 5 drops assumes this is how you purchased it. If you are rich, enough to buy pure chamomile oil then jus add 1 drop.

You will be amazed at how well this treatment works. Do not add extra rose geranium, less is best.

This is a skin brake-out that Mark Antony got when he was fourteen, I was not sure how this happened, nor what it was. What I did was: changed his diet for two weeks to boiled chicken. with no biscuits or liver treats. Day one I put a tiny pinch of bicarbonate of soda in his large water bowl. I changed his bowl with clean water twice daily without adding any bicarbonate of soda. I massaged him every morning on his stomach and the wound, with the above dry skin treatment. I took him for a swim in the ocean, every third day and rinsed him with lukewarm water as soon as we returned home from the beach.

Day one and three I also massaged in some turmeric powder, onto the skin rapture after the Rose Geranium mix had been applied. Use the dry skin oil mixture sparingly on their sore or dry skin.

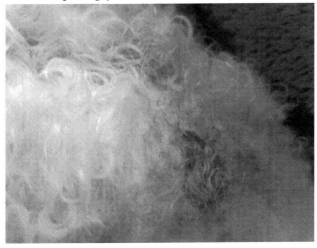

Marks skin after 6 days see next photo. The scab had gone, all the heat and the red inflammation had gone as well.

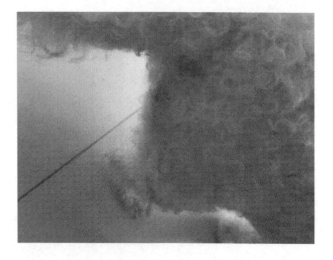

Bicarbonate of Soda. Never add to the Electrolyte mix if your dog has a hernia.

Eye Care

It is very important to take good care of your dogs eyes. They need to have their face rinsed several times a week. They dig with their nose as well as their paws. This causes small dirt particles to go into their eyes. Also, windy days will cause dirt to enter their eyes. If you walk along a beach or river they need to be completely rinsed from ears to paws. Salt and germs can cause all sorts of problems with their skin and eyes.

If your dog has eyes that weep keep the hair cropped very short around their eyes. Add water to a plastic bottle with a nozzle pourer. Gentle squeeze the water over his eyes a few times a day and pat dry with gauze not tissues. If you do not have a nozzle, type bottle then put water in a bowl use some gauze to sponge his eyes.

When his eyes are weeping, the first week every night after dinner bathe his eyes with lukewarm water and pat dry. Place one drop of Chamomile Essential Oil in the bowl of warm water or in the bottle.

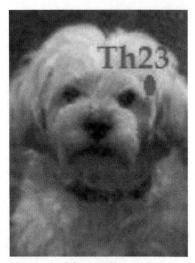

Massage his eyebrow bone. In the acupressure, point TH23.

If eyelids are paralyzed (no blink reflex) the eye's corneal surface may need to be moistened. You can use a sterile lubricant (e.g. Lacrilube, K-Y®), artificial tears, medical saline, or as a last resort even a drop of corn oil or olive oil (if the eye does not appear inflamed). Most antibiotic eye ointments are safe provided they do not contain any kind of cortisone. Or use my Aroma eye mixture

Salmon oil added to their food a few times a week. Just a few drops of Salmon oil will keep their eyes bright and healthy.

Never get shampoo in their eyes.

Grass Seeds in Eyes and Paws.

Prevention Is The Best Cure. Grass seeds do not dissolve in their eyes nor stomachs. If they have one in their paw they may eat it but worst of all the seed can enter into their skin and travel to their heart. I cannot help you fully when it comes to grass seed problems.

1) Regular (DAILY) checking of your dog all over, including in between each and every toe, and especially after a walk

2) Avoid long grass on walks, and keep your grass and weeds short at home

3) Keep long-haired dogs trimmed or clipped, and well groomed, especially around their feet and ears. If trimming them yourself, be mindful of clipping the 'top' off a grass seed, possibly leaving the end still embedded in the skin. This makes it even harder to find.

4) Seek veterinary attention immediately if you suspect a grass seed problem in any location on your dog. Do not expect your groomer to be able to remove these seeds, as they are often too embedded, or require antibiotic treatment once removed. Many times your pet

will need to be sedated to ensure safe grass seed removal, so please be understanding of this.

While walking once through tall grass that was swaying in the wind, Mark Antony got a grass seed in his eye. The vet said it was going to cost several thousands to remove it safely. I was not financially able to spend that kind of money at that time.

I took Mark Antony home and very gently poured olive oil in his eye. I pulled his eyelid over his eyeball. I sat him in my lap and put pressure on his body to hold him firmly in my lap. Then I held pepper corns near his nostril, while holding his eyelid over his eyeball down towards and over his lower lashes. Ever so gently after him sneezing I massaged his eyelid while still over his eyeball. When I let go of his eyelid I very carefully placed the pad of my little finger on the seed and moved it towards the inner corner of his eye. Then with a cotton ball dipped in olive oil carefully flicked the seed out.

Mark Antony had an indent in his eyeball where the seed had been lodged.

I carried Mark Antony to the bathroom. Held his eyelid over his eye again and placed a warm wet face cloth on his eyelid and held it there for about one minute. I then spayed his eyes with "No More Tears" eye drops. Then an hour later massaged his eyelid with Chamomile essential oil. it was 6% Chamomile in Jojoba oil.

It took about six weeks before the indent the seed had made to disappear. Mark Antony did not have any major eye problems from this ordeal. Thanks be to God or my higher power.

Glaucoma.

Here is a great site for you to read about Glaucoma http://veterinaryvision.com/for-veterinarians/emergency-treatment-for-glaucoma/

Eye Care Mix

Buy a 10 ml bottle of Chamomile oil mixed with Jojoba oil.

Massage this into his skin around the eyelid. There is no need to put this mix into his eye the eye will draw in what it needs. Give him eye drops a few times a week, but only if his eyeballs are inflamed.

The important point is to then half an hour to one hour later press a warm wet cloth onto his closed eye. This will stimulate and sooth the eye as well as remove any oil the eye has not taken into the blood vessels. If you are unable to buy the Chamomile and Jojoba oil already mixed together this is what you need.

In a 10 ml dark glass bottle with an eyedropper attached.

Fill with jojoba oil and add 5 drops of Chamomile. But, try to buy the premix.

Fleas

With fleas I could almost fill a book with this problem. Sometimes you think you have the problem licked and other times it drives you crazy. I do not like to be constantly giving my dogs medication to prevent fleas.

One day I gave both my dogs a "Comfortis" tablet Ceasar was fine for a few days but, then back came the fleas. My daughters' dogs are fine when they take their Comfortis tablets. Mark Antony on the other hand - had a terrible reaction to the Comfortis tablet.

His skin broke out in a bright red rash within 20 minutes of having the tablet. He scratched and scratched and ate his hair off in several places. He was whining and was running around in circles.

I prepared a bath with this mix.
- Warm Water
- One tablespoon of Bi-carbonate of soda
- 4 drops of Chamomile Jojoba mix.
- 2 drops Rose Geranium

I sat him in the bath and bathed him using a cup to pour the water over him for 20 minutes.

I then dried him with the blow dryer on a cool setting.
I then sprayed him every hour with this mix:

Dogs Flea Spray

In a spray bottle add:-
2 cups of warm water
Half cup of vinegar
2 drops of Chamomile
1 drop Rose Geranium (optional)
1 drop of Peppermint
2 teaspoon olive oil

Note: once the fleas have gone stop using this mix.

Spraying with this mix will help keep the fleas away
and the dog does not like the taste so it will help
prevent him from chewing at his skin. It is important
to keep his skin cool. If his skin feels hot, you may
have to put him in a vinegar and lukewarm bath every
few hours. The cooler the water the better but if it is
too cold he will fight you to get out sooner than he
should.

For the next few days, I gave him a Chicken ice block
to eat every hour to keep his temperature down. Then

each morning I gave him a small bowl of chicken soup. Each night I gave him his normal 300 grams of chicken casserole. It is important to know how many grams of food your dog should be receiving according to his weight. If you do not know how much food to give your dog, see Feeding Tips below.

You can add 1 extra drop of Peppermint Essential to the above mix to get rid of fleas but not until you have cured his skin rash. The best tablet I found was Capstar. As much as I prefer to use all natural products, I have at times used Capstar, Advantage Plus and Frontline. I usually buy them at the RSPCA opp shop as they are much cheaper there. An opp shop is a secondhand shop run by charity organizations. They sell things very cheaply as they are stocked with donations from the public.

Scratching, scabs and dark specs, or "flea dirt," found on the skin can all be signs that your pet has become the unwitting host for a family of fleas. Whether or not you actually see fleas on your pet, they may be there. Fleas can carry tapeworms, too. If you notice small white rice-like things in your pet's feces or in the hair around his anus, your pet probably has tapeworms, which means he may also have fleas. In extreme cases, an animal may be lethargic and its lips and gums pale.

You have a battle to rid your dog and home of flea infestation. You will need to use a combination of products at the same time to be effective. Plus, you need a lot of patience and a great deal of perseverance. The life cycle of a flea is three to four weeks it will take at least that long to completely; rid your pet and its environment of the enemy.

Different flea control products work in different ways, have varying levels of effectiveness and kill different flea stages (eggs, larvae and/or adults).

Fleas do not like vinegar. That is why it is important to add vinegar to the final rinse when you bath your dog. If you can afford to check with your veterinarian before you begin your war on fleas. Even if you purchase an over-the-counter product, it is wise to consult your veterinarian for any safety concerns.

To assist you with clearing your home of fleas, you may want to consider hiring a professional exterminator (in which case, your veterinarian may be able to recommend one in your area). Dips, shampoos, powders and sprays will usually kill the adult fleas on your pet.

Using a flea comb regularly will help, too. But, more adults may be lurking in your home or yard, and eggs or larvae may be lying in wait, as well. You'll need to rid your house of fleas by vacuuming and washing your pets bedding once a week, and using a disinfectant on washable surfaces and an insecticide or insect growth regulator in cracks and crevices (sometimes foggers are recommended) every two to four weeks.

When using chemical products to control fleas, be very careful. You may be providing too much of a potentially toxic chemical if you use, say, a flea dip and a fogger with the same chemical ingredient. Be sure to empty your vacuum cleaner as soon as you have vacuumed the house and furniture. Spay the vacuum hose and inside the vacuum cleaner with the house flea spray.

House Flea Spray

Keep your home free of lice and flees by spraying this mist under furniture and on your door steps, window sills/ledges and door steps.

> In a spray bottle place 100 ml of alcohol/vinegar . Add :-
>
> 100 ml water
>
> 20 drops of Peppermint oil
>
> 10 Eucalyptus oil
>
> 10 Drops of Lemon oil

Warning: do not spray animals nor yourself with this spay. It is way too strong and will enter your blood stream. Then cause hard balls to form in your liver. Furthermore, you will not know until 20 or more years have passed.

Spay your beds, lounge, carpets, vacuum cleaner hose and filters. Do not use this spray on your pets it far too strong.

Natural Flea Killer For Carpets Is:-.

Bicarbonate of soda and salt.

In a large jar fill with:-
Half bicarbonate of soda and top up with table salt.
Add 10 drops of essential oil of peppermint.
Add 10 drops of rose geranium.

Or buy this on my website.
http://beautyschoolbooks.com/Products.htm

If your pet is an outside pet, you'll need to tackle the yard, too. You can add another 50 drops of peppermint essential oil to the above house spray and spray your yard with the mix. Also, use flea barrier type plants in the garden.

Sunlight kills fleas, so concentrate your efforts in the shady areas of your yard especially. You can spray your yard with insecticide, or you can battle fleas with their natural enemy, nematodes. Nematodes are microscopic worms that kill flea larvae and cocoons. Apply them to your yard once a month until the fleas are gone.

Check with your veterinarian or your pet supply or garden stores to find out more. Nematodes however, can cause other problems with your plants. Only use Nematodes as a last resort for a flea infested yard. This house flea spray, recipe is the best solution for spraying your yard but, it will be expensive, as you will need at least 20 bottles of it for the average size back yard.

I use it just around the house perimeters it takes about three bottles to do the job. I do it at the beginning of Spring then again two weeks later. I then redo it at the beginning of summer and every two weeks during summer. I have lots of peppermint growing as well.

Flea control has reached new levels in recent years. Today, there are products on the market that you can treat your pet with once a month that will help keep those annoying little jumpers away. Insect growth regulators, or IGRs, are safe and act like flea hormones to interrupt the life cycle of the flea, preventing them from maturing into adult fleas. However, I do not like commercial products due to the fact my older dog a Bichon Frise is allergic to them. Yet, for your research, I have added this information.

Lufenuron is one example of an IGR. It inhibits flea egg production, but does not kill adult fleas, so flea bites can still occur. Others, such as imidacloprid and fipronil kill adult fleas and the latter works on ticks as well.

Depending on the product used, you may be giving your pet a pill, spraying his coat or applying a liquid substance to one area of his skin; the substance will spread to cover his body. These treatments are available only from your veterinarian and are given once a month. However, here in Australia the Animal welfare and the RSPCA stores, sell the monthly flea and tick control liquids. Such as:-

Frontline,
Advantage,
Comfortis,
Revolution.

These are great products and they say that they only need to be applied, once a month. Be very careful to use the products as directed; some may be effective for dogs, but toxic to cats. These products although great will not keep the fleas away for the entire month and you should never ever be tempted to use them twice a month. In the height of summer, I do use these products but I also use my Aromatherapy mixes.

Now that you are armored with some information, you can help your pet win the war against fleas.

Flea Seasons

The flea seasons are Spring and Summer. However, in the tropics they can thrive all year round. Less than 20 degrees Celsius there are fewer fleas over 20 degrees Celsius they start to thrive. Try not to walk your dogs in bushy shaded areas.

Plants To Deter Fleas

Using garden plants to get rid of fleas the natural way takes some planning. Flea seasons are Spring and Summer but that doesn't mean fleas are gone from your home or pet. Next spring, pet owners will once again engage in a seasonal battle with fleas. Plan your spring garden to include garden plants that can provide a safe way to get rid of fleas the natural way.

Mints- Peppermint, spearmint, work well around foundations to help repel pests and fleas, keeping them out of the home. We have chocolate mint in front of the house and along sections of our dog pen. A minty aroma is released when the dogs walk through the patch.

Mint is a menacing garden plant, so it's best to put the plants in pots. Pots will keep the mint contained and where you want them to grow. Plant different varieties away from each other to prevent cross pollinating. Mints are inexpensive and easy perennial garden plants to grow and they are hardy- enough to withstand harsh winters.

Place dried leaves in sachet packets and hang around the house or sprinkle in carpets to help get rid of fleas the natural way. Fleas hide in, out of the way places under couches, chairs, along baseboards and beds. Mint doesn't kill fleas, it repels them, but with dedicated use, you can drive fleas out of your home and off your pets.

Do not use peppermint extract because it has alcohol in it. Peppermint oil has the highest level of menthol of all the mints, but any mint will work for flea control.

How To Make Your Own Mint Oil:

Nevertheless, before you go to the trouble of making this mint oil be aware that it does not work as well as the essential oil of peppermint.

If you do not have the Essential oil of mint try this:

Take 1 cup of fresh mint leaves, any variety will work.

Rinse in cool water and pat dry on a paper towel to remove excess water.

Pour 2 cups olive oil, not vegetable oil into a saucepan over medium heat. Vegetable oils contain bleach thanks to naughty manufacturers.

Add the mint leaves, stirring constantly.

Continue stirring for a few minutes until you see the oil beginning to bubble.

Remove from the heat and pour into a bowl, allow to cool to room temperature.

When cooled, add another 2 cups of oil and stir.
Pour oil (and leaves if you want) into a glass container and store in a cool, dark place away from sunlight.

Warning: never put pure mint oil or any other pure essential oil on your pet. Always dilute it in base oil, such as olive oil, sunflower or grape oil. Always dilute first, regardless of which garden plant you used to make the oil mixture.

Note: Homemade mint oil is not anywhere near as strong or effective as the mix I have suggested above made with peppermint essential oil. Use this mixture in the vaporizer.

Aromatherapy Flea Spray

In A Spray Bottle put 100 ml of olive oil
1 drop Peppermint Essential oil
2 drops Rose Geranium.

Walking Spray

Only make and use this if you live in a very bushy area. Less is best. Only do this if you live in a very bushy environment. Shake bottle well. Spray on dogs feet before they go into the yard or you take them for a walk. Avoid their eyes, nose, face and ear area.

In a spray bottle Add.

50 ml of vinegar.

50 ml water

2 drops of peppermint oil.

Spray on dogs feet, {not his paws} and legs before going for his walk.

Note: Use 50 ml of water and 50 mil of vinegar (any kind black or white vinegar}. Keep away from their eyes, as it burns. With this mix it is best just lightly spray their feet and tummy.

For short hair dogs you can replace the alcohol for olive oil. Vinegar is best but you need to be very careful not to get it in their eyes. Also, be sure to add 50% water to the vinegar.

For Large Dogs: Add 2 more drops of Peppermint Essential oil.

Rid Fleas The Natural Way

Rid Fleas The Natural Way With Garden Plants. Some plants are a safe and effective way to get rid of fleas that won't harm any pet, including pets that may wander into my garden.

Catnip is a member of the mint family and is a safe flea control on both cats and dogs. Besides being a natural way to repel fleas, most cats love rolling in it and some will even eat it.

Lavender is a non toxic plant and will repel fleas, moths and mosquitoes. Lavender is a member of the mint family. You can hang bunches of Lavender at your door.

Lemon Grass smells like lemons and repels mosquitoes along with fleas. You can also hang bunches of it at your door.

Chamomile is a small daisy-like flowering plant that is said, to help keep other garden plants be healthy.

Folklore tells us that planting a Chamomile plant next to an unhealthy plant is supposed to help the other plant improve.

Rosemary (the herb) is a member of the mint family and is safe for cats and dogs.

Warning: make sure to plant the Rosemary herb plant and not the Rosemary Pea or Rosemary Bog plant. These two plants Rosemary Pea and Bog Rosemary are toxic to pets.

Sage is the largest plant in the mint family. It grows to around 3 feet tall as a thick bush.

Toxic Flea Plants

Wormwood,

Pennyroyal (Fleabane),

Fleawort,

Tansy,

Rue,

Eucalyptus,

Sweet Bay

Citronella are all listed as garden plants that can be used as a natural way to get rid of fleas, but all of them can be toxic to cats and some are toxic for dogs. I exclude these garden plants and stick with the ones I know are safe for pets. After all, that's the whole idea of using natural flea control.

Some people say not to use essential oils on your pet. They are extremely potent and many, like lavender, eucalyptus, cedar, mint and tea tree, can be toxic to pets even though they are sold as a safe way to get rid of fleas. I often use eucalyptus on my pets but in very tiny amounts.

Essential oils are different from the mint oil described above which is safe for use on pets. However, I have been using Essential oils on pets for over 40 years. Mark Antony is thirteen and he is a healthy dog.

I think people that tell you, not to use them, have not studied Aromatherapy. It could also be that they know most people do not understand how strong they are. That is why you must stick to my recipes and not add extra essential oils to the base oils.

Base oils are Olive, Grape-seed, and Jojoba.

Using garden plants inside and outside the home, to get rid of fleas once and for all, every spring and summer. For a natural way of flea control plants can work, but you have to be committed to winning the battle against fleas and treat pets and their environment. As with anything, you put on your pet, monitor them for signs of any adverse reactions even when using a natural flea control.

In my opinion Pennyroyal is by far the best I have lots of it in pots and places where my dogs cannot get to it. I have it in hanging baskets and pots on tables near my doors. It is a pretty plant and the aroma is amazing. I put a citronella candle in the middle of each pot to deter pets and birds from going near the pots.

Feeding/Water Bowls

Feeding Tips.

1. A good routine is the key, giving set meal times. Never leave food down in the bowl all day as this may lead to fussy eating habits and make weight control hard. Allow 15-20 minutes after putting the food down and remove any leftover. This will also let your local vermin know that of a night there is no food scraps in this house. It is also important to rinse their bowl out at this point.

2. Fussy eaters can be encouraged by adding a small amount of warm water to their dry food. That will bring out the aroma. Be careful not to soak, which will create a mush, as the crunching motion helps clean teeth. A huge number of people think that dry food is all they need to give their dog. Because, the person selling dry food, has not taken the time to explain to you that dry food has lots of added vitamins but does cause the animals' poo to harden. Those added vitamins are all they need each day if you have a healthy dog. What they fail to tell you is that dry food is all you need to give chickens and birds.

Dry food should only be given to dogs a few times a week either as breakfast or added to their evening meal. Dry food usually binds their bowel. Firming up their bowel is often a good thing but if you had to strain to use your bowel, every day you would know something is wrong with your diet.

Another alternative is a teaspoon of 100% Salmon oil to add extra interest as well as promoting healthy joints, bright eyes and a shiny coat. I often sprinkle a little Olive oil and fish oil over their dry food. Mind you, I only give my dogs dry food once a week. They are not keen on it.

3. Be mindful of the amount of treats given, especially around meal times.

4. Always cook the rice separately, wash and drain then store in a separate container. Rice will go rancid within two to three days but the cooked meat or casserole; can be kept in the refrigerator for up to five days. However, I keep three days of their meat or casseroles in the refrigerator and put the rest in the freezer. If giving then Turkey or Duck give them 10% less.

Water Bowls

It is important to have bowls that cannot easily fall over. It is also important to have several bowls, two inside and a few outside. Never put the outside water bowls in the sun.

Be sure to wash them every few days in warm soapy water, then rinse with warm water and refill with cold water. During the winter months, I add a cup of boiling water to the bowl morning and night.

Feeding Quantities

Chicken/Meat or Rice Casserole Quantities

Weight of Dog	Grams per day
1-5kg	35-115 pup 40-130
5-20kg	115-330
20-30kg	330-445
30+kg	445-600

For puppies give them 10% more.

 Never leave lots of dry food out in their bowls. Offer them a small quantity every morning.

1-5kg	¼ cup – ½ cup
5-20kg	½ cup – 1 cup
20-30kg	1 cup – 1 ½ cups
30+kg	2 – 4 cups

Then during the day give them a bone and a piece of dried beef/chicken or live treat. I give my dogs one Smacko.

Grooming

See Brushing and Bathing

Gums = Health Check

There are many reasons why you should constantly be aware of the state and colour of your dogs gums. If you do not know what colour they are normally, you will not know how to check his health condition, when he becomes sick.

You will not know if he is dehydrated and in a dangerous situation.

At least once a week clean his teeth and check the colour of his gums and how quickly the blood returns when you press his gums.

Press the gum above the front teeth. The gum should go whitish under your finger pressure and as you release, one second later his gum should turn back to its normal colour. If it is slow to return the dog is in trauma.

The appearance of the gums is very informative. If the gums are:-

Blue, the dog lacks oxygen.

White, the dog has lost blood either internally or externally.

Purple or gray and there is a slow capillary refill, the dog is probably in shock.

Bright red, she may be fighting a systemic infection or may have been exposed to a toxin.

Some dogs have black-pigmented gums, which can make assessment difficult. For these dogs, you need to examine the pink tissue on the inside of the lower eyelid by gently pulling the eyelid down. In this case, you can only observe the colour of the tissue you cannot perform the capillary refill test but colours mean the same thing in gums and inner eyelids.

Pet's Elimination Habits: Hard Poo

The problem could be no more complicated than a lack of fiber in the diet or inadequate water consumption; it may be a more serious cause.

Constipation is when he either has difficulty pooping (and feces produced are dry and hard) or he is not using his bowels at all.

If solid waste stays in your dog's colon too long, all the moisture in it will be absorbed and stools will become dry, hard, and difficult to pass. The food turns to a substance like timber.

Earlier this year Mark Antony had not eliminated his bowel for three days. I put olive oil up his back passage and added it to his water bowl. He was not eating and I was very concerned.

I gave him an enema and that did not help. So I gave him some boiled prunes with olive oil. I had to force them down his throat and gave him another enema. I gave him another enema, and then took him to the beach for a run, he was not very interested in running and playing with other dogs but being down the beach for over an hour did force him to walk more than he would have on our usual run around the block. He still did not use his bowel. So after being home for an hour I gave him another enema put olive oil in the enema and took him for another walk. Finally, he went without too much straining. The first few bowel movements where very hard and had a little blood with the poo. His poo was like small pieces of timber.

As we continued to walk he did a lovely big softer poo with no blood. The prunes had worked. For the next few days he had chicken ice blocks and chicken casserole with a teaspoon of salmon oil added. I did not give him any biscuits nor his liver treats. I did give him some raw bones to chew on but he was not very interested in food.

When the situation is left untreated, your dog's large intestine will actually stretch to the point where it can no longer do its job effectively. This is a chronic condition known as mega-colon, and is actually more common in cats than dogs.

Your goal should be to prevent your pets from ever having such chronic and longstanding bowel issues.

Whether you take your dog out to do his business or he goes out his doggy door into the backyard at will, it is important to keep an eye on his elimination habits. The quantity of urine and feces, the colour, texture, smell, and the presence of mucus or blood – are all indicators of how well your pet's body is functioning.

What leaves your dog's body is warns if there is the first sign of a problem with his health. it is important if you don't accompany your dog out to potty, that you regularly monitor the areas of your yard or property where he does his business.

Most dogs with constipation will look like they are trying to go need to go but don't go. If after several minutes of hunching and straining, your pooch has produced either nothing or a small, hard something, you can safely assume he is constipated. This is especially true if the problem lasts more than a day or two. You may notice your constipated dog appears bloated. He may be in some pain as well, especially during the act of trying unsuccessfully to poop. If he's able to pass stool, it may have an odd colour – usually darker than normal. You may notice mucus or blood or other oddities you've never noticed before.

If the situation persists, your dog may have episodes of vomiting. He could lose his appetite and begin to drop weight. He may appear listless. Ideally, the situation won't get this far before action is taken. That is why it's important to regularly monitor not only what goes into your dog's body, but also what comes out of it. However, Mark Antony lost 2 kilo within a few days.

Causes of Constipation

There are many potential causes of constipation. They all fall into one of three categories as follows:

1. Interluminal (micro calcifications) causes involve partial or complete obstruction on the inside of the colon, brought on by ingestion of matter than can't be digested, as well as tumors.

2. Extraluminal (tissue pressure) causes occur outside the colon and contribute to obstructive constipation, for example, a narrowed pelvis resulting from a pelvic fracture, or tumors growing in the pelvic cavity that compress the bowel from the outside.

3. Intrinsic causes are neuromuscular in nature and can result from pelvic or lumbar nerve injury or diseases like hypothyroidism or hypocalcaemia.

A partial list of causes includes:-

1. •Dehydration, not enough dietary fiber, lack of exercise
2. •Infected anal glands or a hip or pelvic injury that causes pain during defecation
3. •Intestinal obstruction, including tumors
4. •Neuromuscular disorders involving abnormalities or injury to the nerves or muscles of the colon

5. •The effects of surgery, some medications, and iron supplements
6. •Stress brought on by a change in routine or surroundings
7. •Swallowing a foreign object like a piece of cloth, part of a shoe, or rocks

One of the most frequent causes of constipation in dogs is dehydration. If you suspect your pup is constipated or you have noticed dry, hard stools when he is able to go, it's important to monitor his water intake.

To calculate how much water your dog needs. Remember, very active pets need more water, and every dog's requirements increase in hot weather.

Make sure your pup always has easy access to clean, fresh water, and if you suspect she's not drinking enough, measure it out into her bowl to keep better track of her actual consumption.

Depending on what you feed your pet – especially if you feed raw or cooked food prepared at home, or a canned commercial formula -- she should be getting some of the moisture her body needs from her meals. If you feed dry kibble to your dog, your dog, will need to get most of her water from her water bowl exclusively, which I do not recommend unless you can't afford to feed a more species-appropriate form of food.

 If your dog ingests a non-food foreign object, which dogs are known to do, or even a big chunk of bone, it can lodge in his bowel and cause an obstruction around which stools cannot pass. If your dog is having trouble pooping and he has been known to swallow things he should not, my advice is to contact your vet if the situation doesn't resolve in a day or two.

If you are unable to get to the vet give your dog a spoon of cod liver oil or olive oil. Add 1 tablespoon of milk to his food and a teaspoon of olive oil. Chances are he is not interested in food so you will need to put the oil and milk in his mouth. Administer very slowly as you do not want it to go down the wrong way. He may suck on a ice block made up oil and milk. You will also need to give him an enema. See Dogs Enema

If you know for a fact your pet has ingested something large that could create an obstruction, don't delay as this can develop quickly into a very serious, even fatal, problem.

Intact male dogs, especially as they age, can develop enlarged prostates which compress the bowel, creating pencil thin stools or even an obstruction. This problem can usually be resolved by having your pet neutered.

Hernias in your dog's rectum in the area next to the anus can cause constipation. The hernia bulges into the rectum, closing off passage of stool. Hernias usually require surgery to repair.

Some dogs have insufficient muscle tone or neuromuscular disorders that impede their body's ability to efficiently - move waste through the colon. Stool that stays too long in the bowel loses moisture and hardens, making it even more difficult for the dog to go. This can become a vicious cycle, because the more difficult or painful it is to go, the more likely the dog is to develop a habit of avoiding elimination.

When to Worry

If dog develops constipation that does not resolve in a day or two, it's smart to be concerned. There are potentially life-threatening causes of constipation in canines, so it is important to keep a close eye on a constipated pet and seek medical help if things do not improve quickly.

If your dog's constipation resolves in a day or two but recurs, again, it's time to see your veterinarian. A recurrence indicates the problem may be more complicated and require either medical intervention or permanent changes to your dog's diet or lifestyle.

Chronic constipation is known as obstipation. This is a very unfortunate situation, in which a dog is unable to empty his bowels without outside help. The colon becomes enlarged, as it retains a growing volume of hard stool.

A dog with constipation will be extremely uncomfortable and try often but unsuccessfully to poop. Without intervention, he will lose his appetite, become lethargic and begin to vomit.

Depending on the severity of the situation, intervention can mean IV fluids for hydration and an enema to clear the colon. It can mean the dog must be fully anesthetized for a manual cleanout. Often, a second round is required to remove stool that was packed into inaccessible areas of the bowel during the first procedure. Surgery is always required in intractable cases.

What to Do and What Not to Do

Constipation: A constipated dog spends longer than usual defecating (eliminating, pooping), and the resultant stools are small, round, and hard. You can bet that if your dog is constipated, he is uncomfortable.

One of the main causes of constipation is insufficient water, often coupled with too much time between outdoor potty breaks. The walks are short. Dogs need to run free at least four times a week preferably daily.

All too often, I see people taking their dogs for nice slow walks on the lead every day. Dogs do need to be allowed to run freely and smell different smells. Here in Australia we have plenty of dog free areas that are safe and loads of fully fenced dog free play areas.

How To Help Your Dog

Make sure your dog always has plenty of fresh water to flush her intestinal tract.

Add vegetables to your dog diet.

Give plenty of exercise, either walking or playing fetch or anything, which will stimulate her bowels. Offer canned pumpkin in its pureed form (not pumpkin pie filling)

Give one teaspoon of salmon or olive oil for a dog but much less for a puppy.

Offer a small bowl of milk.

There are laxatives "Lactulose" is one formulated specifically for pets.

Using a warm (not hot) moist wash cloth, gently apply slight pressure on his tummy while stroking downward toward the anus. This action mimics the natural way a mother dog uses her tongue to help her pup to eliminate trapped gas while encouraging the elimination of waste and urine.

If you will be away from home for a long time, arrange for a neighbor or a professional pet sitter to let your dog out to relieve himself. Never withhold water from your pet as this could set him up for kidney problems and other behavioral issues. Prevent constipation by adding vegetables to his diet. Many people use a combination of cut green beans mixed with wetted dry dog food.

Milk or ice cream will often help the constipation problem as dogs that are reluctant to drink water will most often drink milk if offered and most love an ice cream. Offer a small bowlful and let him lap it up. He may initially have a runny stool but it should solve the constipation problem. Ice-cream should not be given as a treat but, it is OK on the odd occasion when they need to soften their bowel movement.

The reason it will cause a runny poo is they are actually allergic to milk.

Before attempting anything, remember how a mother dog helps her young offspring to eliminate waste.

Using her tongue, she gently but, firmly licks in a downward motion from the bottom of his buttocks.

If the pup is very small, use a moist cotton ball instead of the cloth. The warmth of the cotton ball or cloth, combined with the gentle downward motion should help your puppy eliminate, ending his constipation problem. If this does not work, read on.

Dogs Enema

An enema can be given, using a #8 feeding tube, attached to a syringe (without the needle of course), filled with approximately 2 to 5 cc's of warm (not hot) water (the amount depends on the size of the puppy.)

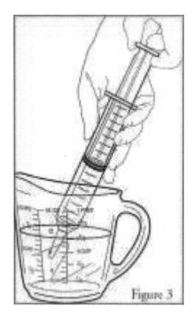

Figure 3

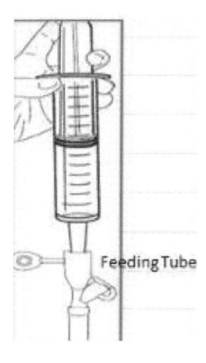

After filling the syringe attach it to a feeding tube. Sit with the dog.

Hold his tail up.

Place some Aloe Vera gel in his rectum.

Now gently push the feeding tube in.

Press the Syringe top so the liquid goes into his bum hole.

Gently remove the tube.

It will be best now if he plays outside or is kept in an area that has no carpet.

In about an hours time take him for a walk.

You may need to repeat this process again in about four hours time.

You can use Microlax on dogs, which you buy from the local Chemist/Drug Store. Just give him a tiny piece. Ask your Pharmacist for some advise on the quantity or speak with a veterinary or his nurse. Dogs have various responses to various products , so air on the side of caution. Less is best.

Foods That Keep Him Regular

Psyllium husk powder: 1/2 teaspoon per 4.55 kilo/10 pounds of body weight 1-2 times daily on food.

Ground dark green leafy veggies: 1 teaspoon per 4.55 kilo/10 pounds of body weight 1-2 times daily with food.

Coconut fiber: 1 teaspoon per 4.5 kilo /10 pounds of body weight 1-2 times daily on food.

Canned 100 percent pumpkin: 1 teaspoon per 4.55 kilo /10 pounds of body weight 1-2 times daily on food. I like to add raw pumpkin pieces to their food once a week. But, if they are constipated I boil it and add to their meat.

Organic apple cider vinegar is a bit of a natural wonder drug, in that it can alleviate a wide variety of conditions in both people and pets. It is well known, to improve digestion, including relieving constipation.

1/4 teaspoon per 4.55 kilo /10 pounds of body weight added to your dog's food 1-2 times daily.

Aloe juice (not the topical gel): 1/4 teaspoon per 4.55 kilo/10 pounds of body weight 1-2 times daily on food.

The plant Aloe Vera is my choice. I scrape out the inner jelly and add to their food and also apply to the inside of their rectum.

Chiropractic, acupuncture/pressure and massage. All three of these natural modalities have been proven to help with chronic constipation in pets.

Massage GV14 and GB30.

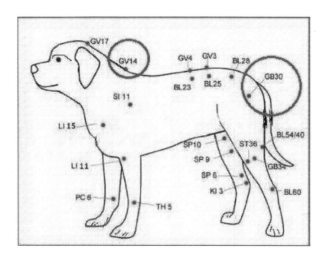

Acupuncture Treatment

Dogs treated with electro acupuncture (EA) combined with Chinese herbal medicine for a period of six months. As a result of the acupuncture and herbal medicine therapy, the dog showed significant improvement in spinal posture, proprioception, and mobility. The acupuncture points used were UB18, UB22, UB23, UB25, UB26, UB27, UB28, UB37, UB60, GB30, GB31, GB34, Du14, St36, and K1. Electro acupuncture was set to pairs of points at 30 Hz for 10 minutes followed by 80-120 Hz for another

10 minutes. In addition, vitamin B12 was injected into acupuncture points UB23, GB30, St36 and K1. The dog received electro acupuncture twice weekly for a period of one month followed by electro acupuncture once every two weeks for five months.

The herbal formula Du Huo Ji Sheng Tang for 6 months in a semi-solid form mixed with honey was administered. Additional care included swimming. In this procedure, the dog was placed in a bathtub twice a week for 20 minutes while the owner stabilized the dog. The dog was encouraged to swim with the feet "barely" touching the bottom of the bathtub. Other additional care included vitamins and supplements including: omega-3 oils, vitamin E, vitamin B complex, glucosamine and chondroitin sulfate.

Results

The dog improved with a "restoration of normal walk, defecation and urination" as measured after six months of therapy. The back pain was measured to have completely resolved and proprioception normalized. The ambulatory parapesis condition improved and the thoracolumbar disc disease decreased from a level V to a level II.

Have a look at this site:

http://www.dovehealth.com/uncategorized/dog-acupressure-treatments/

Do Not

Please don't give your dog any human laxatives meant for humans or stool softener without consulting your veterinarian. There are laxatives "Lactulose" is one formulated specifically for pets. And Microlax although for humans is safe for dogs.

High fiber grains meant for humans. Don't attempt to resolve your dog's constipation with grains, cereals or other high fiber people foods without consulting your holistic veterinarian first.

Remember your dog is a carnivore. Grains are not a natural part of his diet and could make a bad situation worse.

Mineral Oil Dangers.

Please don't give your animals mineral oil. It's not effective, and it can be inhaled into the lungs, causing permanent damage. It will not dissolve in an animal nor humans body.

Home-Made Enemas.

Put a cup of warm water and a pinch of salt and one teaspoon of olive oil in a mug/jug. Use a pipette to draw the mix up. Put some olive oil up his back passage. Smooth some olive oil on the outside of the pipette. Now gently insert the pipette in as far as it will go without pushing too much. Some dogs will resist and you can tear the delicate skin inside their bum. So, do it with love and take your time. When the pipette is in, squeeze the mixture into his back passage. Then take him for a walk. You may have to do this several times with three to four hour intervals for a few days.

Dogs Do Eat Poo

It is wise to discourage your dog from eating poo even though it is a natural act for them. If the problem persists after a few months of you saying in a firm voice "no" then you will need to research the problem or seek help. Never crawl at your dog if he does his poo in the house that will encourage him to eat it so he does not get into trouble.

Take him for a routine walk of a night when he does poo, on the footpath pick it up and say good boy, very good boy and give him a pat. When you get home and have disposed of the poo bag, put some paper down where he usually likes to poo. When he does his poo on the paper, reward him.

Dogs Acupressure Points

Press these points with your pointy finger and circulate the point for a few seconds then move to the next point and do the same. Massaging these points will help with all kinds of ailments and
I strongly urge you to buy a good book on these pressure points.

When your dog is constipated massage points GV14 to GB30 and massage his tummy.

I actually tried to buy these charts and emailed the owners of this work so I could give you more information. But, I had no luck. I have put there site below so you can try.

This chart is a free download at

Yes, you will have to copy and paste that entire http, that I have highlighted into your web browser address bar.

http://rowandogblog.blogspot.com.au/p/normal-0-false-false-false.html

Foods That Poison Dogs

This information on foods that are poisons to dogs was from ASPCA pet-care

http://www.aspca.org/Pet-care/virtual-pet-behaviorist/dog-articles/foods-that-are-hazardous-to-dogs

Most dogs love food, and they are especially attracted to what they see. While sharing the occasional tidbit with your dog is fine, it is important to be aware that some foods can be very dangerous to dogs. Take caution to make sure your dog never gets access to the foods below. Even if you don't give him table scraps, your dog might eat something that is hazardous to his health if he raids kitchen counters, cupboards and trash cans. For advice on teaching your dog not to steal food, please see our article, Counter Surfing and Garbage Raiding.

Avocado

Avocados are toxic to a number of animals, including horses, rabbits, fish and mice. The toxic effects are due to the compound persin, an oil-soluble toxin found in specialized cells (idioblasts) within the avocado fruit, as well as in its skin. In some animals, persin causes damage to the heart muscle cells, leading to heart failure. In other species, it causes an inflammation of the mammary glands.

The toxicity of avocado to dogs is under question. Although one case report indicated that two dogs developed fatal heart failure after ingesting a "large amount" of avocados, most dogs who eat avocado suffer no serious injury.

However, until the susceptibility of dogs to persin is further investigated, it is safest to avoid feeding avocado to your dog. In addition to the possibility he'll have a bad reaction to the fruit itself, your dog might swallow the pit, which could result in blockage within his digestive tract—and that might require surgery.

Bread Dough

Raw bread dough made with live yeast can be hazardous if ingested by dogs. When raw dough is swallowed, the warm, moist environment of the stomach provides an ideal environment for the yeast to multiply, resulting in an expanding mass of dough in the stomach. Expansion of the stomach may be severe enough to decrease blood flow to the stomach wall, resulting in the death of tissue. Additionally, the expanding stomach may press on the diaphragm, resulting in breathing difficulty. Perhaps more importantly, as the yeast multiplies, it produces alcohols that can be absorbed, resulting in alcohol intoxication. Affected dogs may have distended abdomens and show signs such as a lack of coordination, disorientation, stupor and vomiting (or attempts to vomit).

In extreme cases, coma or seizures may occur and could lead to death from alcohol intoxication. Dogs showing mild signs should be closely monitored, and dogs with severe abdominal distention or dogs who are so inebriated that they can't stand up should be monitored by a veterinarian until they recover.

Chocolate

Chocolate intoxication is most commonly seen around certain holidays—like Easter, Christmas, Halloween and Valentine's Day—but it can happen any time dogs have access to products that contain chocolate, such as chocolate candy, cookies, brownies, chocolate baking goods, cocoa powder and cocoa shell-based mulches.

The compounds in chocolate that cause toxicosis are caffeine and theobromine, which belong to a group of chemicals called methylxanthines. The rule of thumb with chocolate is "the darker it is, the more dangerous it is." White chocolate has very few methylxanthines and is of low toxicity. Dark baker's chocolate has very high levels of methylxanthines, and plain, dry unsweetened cocoa powder contains the most concentrated levels of methylxanthines. Depending on the type and amount of chocolate ingested, the signs seen can range from vomiting, increased thirst, abdominal discomfort and restlessness to severe agitation, muscle tremors, irregular heart rhythm, high body temperature, seizures and death.

Dogs showing more than mild restlessness should be seen by a veterinarian immediately.

Alcohol

Ethanol (Also Known as Ethyl Alcohol, Grain Alcohol or Drinking Alcohol)

Dogs are far more sensitive to ethanol than humans are. Even ingesting a small amount of a product containing alcohol can cause significant intoxication. Dogs may be exposed to alcohol through drinking alcoholic drinks, such as beer, wine or mixed drinks (those with milk, like White Russians and "fortified" egg-nogs, are especially appealing to dogs), alcohol-containing elixirs and syrups, and raw yeast bread dough (please see the above section on bread dough). Alcohol intoxication commonly causes vomiting, loss of coordination, disorientation and stupor. In severe cases, coma, seizures and death may occur. Dogs showing mild signs of alcohol intoxication should be closely monitored, and dogs who are so inebriated, that they can't stand up should be monitored by a veterinarian until they recover.

Grapes and Raisins

Grapes and raisins have recently been associated with the development of kidney failure in dogs. At this time, the exact cause of the kidney failure isn't clear, nor is it clear why some dogs can eat these fruits without harm, while others develop life-threatening problems after eating even a few grapes or raisins.

Some dogs eat these fruits and experience no ill effects—but then eat them later on and become very ill. Until the cause of the toxicosis is better identified, the safest course of action is to avoid feeding grapes or raisins to your dog.

Dogs experiencing grape or raisin toxicosis usually develop vomiting, lethargy or diarrhea within 12 hours of ingestion. As signs progress, dogs become increasingly lethargic and dehydrated, refuse to eat and may show a transient increase in urination followed by decreased or absent urination in later stages. Death due to kidney failure may occur within three to four days, or long-term kidney disease may persist in dogs who survive the acute intoxication. Successful treatment requires prompt veterinary treatment to maintain good urine flow.

Hops

Cultivated hops used for brewing beer have been associated with potentially life-threatening signs in dogs that have ingested them. Both fresh and spent (cooked) hops have, been implicated in poisoning dogs. Affected dogs develop an uncontrollably high body temperature (often greater than 108 degrees Fahrenheit), which results in damage to and failure of multiple organ systems. Dogs poisoned by hops become restless, pant excessively, and may have muscle tremors and seizures. Prompt veterinary intervention is necessary to prevent death in these dogs. Beer is made with Hops and so are many other items.

Macadamia Nuts

Although macadamia nut toxicosis is unlikely to be fatal in dogs, it can cause very uncomfortable symptoms that may persist for up to 48 hours. Affected dogs develop weakness in their rear legs, appear to be in pain, may have tremors and may develop a low grade fever. Fortunately, these signs will gradually subside over 48 hours, but dogs experiencing more than mild symptoms can benefit from veterinary care, which may include intravenous fluid therapy and pain control.

Moldy Foods

A wide variety of molds grow on food. Some produce toxins called tremorgenic mycotoxins, which can cause serious or even life-threatening problems if ingested by dogs. Unfortunately, it's not possible to determine whether a particular mold is producing tremorgenic mycotoxins, so the safest rule of thumb is to avoid feeding dogs moldy food. In other words, if you wouldn't eat it, neither should your dog.

Promptly remove any trash or moldy debris (road-kill, fallen walnuts or fruit, etc.) from your dog's environment to prevent him from eating it. The signs of tremorgenic mycotoxin poisoning generally begin as fine muscle tremors that progress to very coarse total-body tremors and, finally, convulsions that can lead to death in severe cases. Left untreated, these tremors can last for several weeks. Fortunately, they usually respond well to appropriate veterinary treatment.

Onions and Garlic

Be sure to read this entire section on Garlic and Onions.

Note: I can seldom give Mark Antony garlic and it does not help with his fleas. I have given Ceasar garlic when he had parvovirus and a bad does of the fleas.

Garlic's medicinal properties

There are many health benefits to feeding garlic. Here are some things you might not know about this healthy herb:

Garlic is a natural antibiotic and won't affect the good bacteria in the gut which are needed for digestion and immune health.

- Garlic is antifungal
- Garlic is antiviral

- Garlic boosts the immune system
- Garlic makes dogs less desirable to fleas
- Garlic is anti-parasitic

What kind of garlic?

With that said, I have researched Garlic for dogs as Mark Antony comes out in a rash when I add it to his food. Ceasar on the other hand does not. The food scientist believe you should not add onion or garlic to food that you are going to store over night or store for a few days. I myself have a weak stomach and if I eat leftover food with onion or garlic in it two days after storing I become sick. Therefore, my belief is do not give dogs garlic unless they are ill and need an antibiotic.

Also, use the food that contains garlic within 10 hours. The other option is to add crushed raw garlic to a sick dogs meal each day for a few days and never ever give dogs onion.

All close members of the onion family (shallots, onions, garlic, scallions, etc.) contain compounds that can damage dogs' red blood cells if ingested in sufficient quantities. A rule of thumb is "the stronger it is, the more toxic it is." Garlic tends to be more toxic than onions, on an ounce-for-ounce basis.

While it's uncommon for dogs to eat enough raw onions and garlic to cause serious problems, exposure to concentrated forms of onion or garlic, such as dehydrated onions, onion soup mix or garlic powder, may put dogs at risk of toxicosis.

The damage to the red blood cells caused by onions and garlic generally doesn't become apparent until three to five days after a dog eats these vegetables. Affected dogs may seem weak or reluctant to move, or they may appear to tire easily after mild exercise. Their urine may be orange-tinged to dark red in colour. These dogs should be examined by a veterinarian immediately. In severe cases, blood transfusions may be needed.

Xylitol

Xylitol is a non-caloric sweetener that is widely used in sugar-free gum, as well as in sugar-free baked products. In humans, xylitol does not affect blood sugar levels, but in dogs, ingestion of xylitol can lead to a rapid and severe drop in blood sugar levels. Dogs may develop disorientation and seizures within 30 minutes of ingesting xylitol-containing products, or signs may be delayed for several hours. Some dogs that ingest large amounts of xylitol develop liver failure, which can be fatal. All dogs ingesting xylitol-containing products should be examined by a veterinarian immediately.

Immunization/vaccinations

I keep my dogs well vaccinated until they are two years old. By then my healthy dog program has set in and I stop with the recommended veterinary doses.

At 6-8 weeks of age puppies should receive their first vaccination; this is temporary and needs to be followed up with another one at 12 weeks. After the 12 week vaccination you can then take your puppy out in public areas.

Although vaccination has the potential to protect pets against life-threatening diseases, vaccination is not without its risks. Recently, there has been some controversy regarding the duration of protection and timing of vaccination, as well as the safety and necessity of certain vaccines.

Vaccination is a procedure that has risks and benefits, that need to be considered for each dog, relative to his lifestyle and health.

Vaccines help prepare the body's immune system to fight the invasion of disease-causing organisms. Vaccines contain antigens, which look like the disease-causing organism to the immune system but do not actually cause disease. When the vaccine is introduced to the body, the immune system is mildly stimulated. If a dog is ever exposed to the real disease, his immune system is now prepared to recognize and fight it off entirely or reduce the severity of the illness.

Bottom line-vaccines are very important in managing the health of your dog. That said, not every dog needs to be vaccinated against every disease. It is very important to work out the best vaccination protocol that's right for your dog. Factors that should be examined include age, medical history, environment, travel habits and lifestyle. Most vets highly recommend administering core vaccines to healthy dogs.

Core Vaccines

In 2006, the American Animal Hospital Association's Canine Task Force published a revised version of guidelines regarding canine vaccinations. The guidelines divide vaccines into three categories-core, non-core and not recommended.

Core vaccines are considered vital to all dogs based on risk of exposure, severity of disease or transmissibility to humans. Canine parvovirus, distemper, canine hepatitis and rabies are considered core vaccines.

Non-core vaccines

Are given to your dog depending on the dogs exposure to risk. These include vaccines against:-

Bordetella
Bronchisepticato
Borrelia burgdorferi
Leptospira bacteria.

Your veterinarian can determine what vaccines are best for your dog. But watch the dog closely for a few days. Ceasar is almost always fine but Mark Antony is more often than not sick after injections. Therefore, I do not vaccinate my Dogs as often as the Vets say I should.

For more information have a look at these websites:-

http://pets.webmd.com/dogs/guide/routine-vaccinations-puppies-dogs

http://www.vetwest.com.au/pet-library/caring-for-your-dog-vaccinations-worming-flea-heartworm-feeding

Vet West is a good site to get quick answers from. They give short to the point answers.

However, veterinarians make money from vaccinations so it is best that you work it out for yourself. As I, have stated above the first two years vaccinations are vitally important. I myself never get the flue or other sicknesses that other people seem to get all the time.

In my home I vaporize essential oils every few days. I replace chemical cleaners with vinegar, bicarbonate of soda and essential oils.

Lethargy Tired Dog

Happy healthy dogs do sleep a lot. When they get up in the morning they have lots of energy and need to play or run about for a while. Then again about 2 pm, they need to have some fun. After their evening meal, they will want to go for a wonder or a walk. Other than that, they usually sleep.

You only need to worry when the dog no longer gets excited about going outside with you. Should this occur check his vital signs as per my section "Daily Health Check" If everything seems to be as it should, take him to the dog free area for some play time. This area should also have a grassy area where he can roam as he may need to eat some grass.

If gums are slow to return to normal when you press them, then you need to take him to the Veterinary. But sometimes they can just be a little off colour, just like us.

Nose

There is a common belief that a healthy dog has a cold, wet nose and a sick dog has a hot, dry nose is FALSE.

The dogs' nose temperatures fluctuate day to day, even hour to hour. It's hard to say exactly why (it could be the environment or it could be what they've been up to recently). But, a dog can be perfectly healthy and have a warm, dry nose. A dog can be really sick (think heart disease or critically injured) and have a cold, moist nose.

The moistness of your dog's nose is also not an indicator of health. However, dogs can have moist noses because they're healthy, and they can have moist noises when they have a nasal disease. It's just not a reliable sign. Better indicators of a dog's health are symptoms such as not eating, not drinking, or behaving oddly.

Make a Dogs Coat.

The size of your dog will dictate the amount of fabric you will need. You can buy the pattern, it is by KWIK SEW. However, if you are smart enough you can make the pattern. Measure the length of your dog, for the body of the coat and then two and a half times the length of your dog for the wrap around. If you make it in felt you can cut a fringe around the edges. Felt is water repellant but, I sprayed mine with silicone spray. Most fabric stores sell it. If your dog has long or fluffy hair then it is best to glue some satin fabric to the inside of the coat. The satin will prevent his hair or fur from knotting up.

With this design all you need is fabric and scissors.

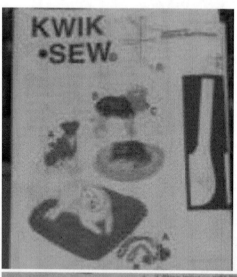

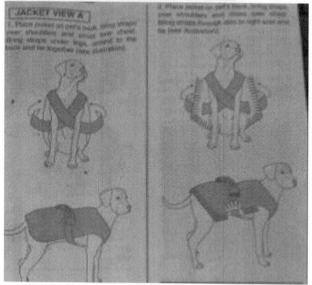

Panting

Unlike humans, dogs don't sweat; they regulate their body temperature through panting- using their tongue and airway as a cooling mechanism. Dogs that are unable to move air efficiently are not only more likely to suffer heat stress; they're also less likely to move enough air into their bodies to oxygenate their blood efficiently. This helps explain why snore-prone breeds can suffer from chronic fatigue.

Dogs that endure a lifetime of poor breathing can end up getting hiatus hernias, which can be life threatening. So yes, something as seemingly harmless as snoring can instigate other health troubles that create a domino effect down a dangerous path. But then again, the same can be said, for humans who snore due to something like obstructive sleep apnea, which can trigger respiratory and circulatory distress farther down the line.

My dog Ceasar pants very hard and fast of a night while he is sleeping. I need to massage him and give him some smelling salts to settle him down.

Smelling Salts For Anxious Dogs.

In a small cotton bag or small cotton sock, place a few tablespoons of sea salt. If you have dried Lavender flowers place a tablespoon of the Lavender in the bag as well, Add:-

4 drops of Chamomile
4 drops of Lavender

Place the bag under his nose but not on his nose this will clear his airways and induce a peaceful heart rhythm. Then place this bag in an airtight jar. It will keep for 18 months.

Parvo Virus

The parvovirus is a severe and highly contagious disease of dogs. The virus has a tendency to attack rapidly reproducing cells, such as those lining the gastrointestinal tract.

The virus is shed - in large amounts in the stools of acutely infected dogs for up to several weeks following infection. The disease is transmitted by oral contact with infected feces. Parvo can be carried on the dog's hair and feet, as well as on contaminated crates, shoes, and other objects. When the dog licks the fecal material off hair, feet, or anything that came in contact with infected feces, he acquires the disease.

If an infected dog bites your dog, the parvovirus will be injected into your dog within minutes.

Parvo affects dogs of all ages, but most cases occur in puppies 6 to 20 weeks of age. Doberman Pinschers and Rottweiler appear to acquire the infection more readily and experience more severe symptoms. The reason for lower resistance in these breeds is unknown. Dehydration develops rapidly.

You can suspect parvo in all pups with the abrupt onset of vomiting and diarrhea. The most efficient way to diagnose parvo is to identify either the virus or virus antigens in stools. An in-office blood serum test (ELISA) is available for rapid veterinary diagnosis. False negatives do occur. Virus isolation techniques are more precise, but require an outside laboratory.

Parvo Treatment:

Dogs with this parvo disease require intensive veterinary management. In all but the mildest cases, hospitalization is essential to correct dehydration and electrolyte imbalances. Intravenous fluids and medications to control vomiting and diarrhea are often required. More severe cases may require blood plasma transfusions and other intensive care.

Puppies and dogs should not eat or drink until the vomiting has stopped. But require fluid support during that time. This can take three to five days. Antibiotics are prescribed to prevent septicemia and other bacterial complications, which are the usual cause of death.

The outcome depends upon the virulence of the specific strain of parvovirus, the age and immune status of the dog, and how quickly the treatment is - started. Most pups who are under good veterinary care recover without complications. But some vets although charming are not all that caring. You need to keep a close eye on your dogs progress;

Parvo Prevention:

Thoroughly clean and disinfect the quarters of infected animals. Parvo is an extremely hardy virus that resists most household cleaners and survives on the premises for months. The most effective disinfectant is household bleach in a 1:32 dilution.

The bleach must be left on the contaminated surface for 20 minutes before being rinsed.

If your dog rolls in the poo while out walking as some dogs love to do give him a bath immediately. Then apply some of the flea spray. The fleas spray is also a disinfectant. See "Dogs Flea Spray"

Prevention Is Better Than Cure

House Hold cleaner And vapourizers

I love the many uses of vinegar and bicarbonate of soda for cleaning. Keep you and your family, plus your pets safe by using homemade cleaners.

Vaporizers filled with essential oils are the Guardian Angel to every home.

In An Oil Burner I Place:-

1 cup of warm water
1 drop of lemon to cleanse the air in my home.
1 drops of eucalyptus to warn off harmful bacterial

2 drops of orange oil to excite my happiness chemicals.

In The Evening

I place just 6 drops of lavender with the warm water in the oil burner to promote a quiet and peaceful environment.

"Olfactory cilia" is a fancy way of saying "nose hairs," but is important to distinguish between the macroscopic nose hairs near the opening of the nostrils, and the microscopic hairs in the olfactory epithelium, the part of the nose which traps smells and communicates them to the brain. The microscopic olfactory cilia play a very important role in the perception of smell, and they perform several other functions for the nose as well.

Properly speaking, the visible nose hair is just hair, not cilia. Cilia are specialized biological structures which closely resemble hair, but on a much smaller scale. The nose hair near the front of the nose helps to trap particulate matter, preventing harmful materials from entering the nasal passages and defending the body from potential sources of infection. Because of this important function, many doctors do not recommend trimming nose hair, no matter how aesthetically displeasing it may be.

The olfactory cilia inside the nose line the mucus membranes of the nose, and unlike most other cilia in the body, they are non-motile, remaining stationary in the nose rather than wiggling around in the mucus like the cilia which line the trachea and intestines do. As smells enter the nose, they dissolve in the mucus and come into contact, with the olfactory cilia.

The cilia in turn transmit the smell to the olfactory nerve, which passes the information on to the brain. This process can be lightning-fast, as anyone who has ever walked past sewage treatment plant can tell you.

Photo under microscope of olfactory cilia.

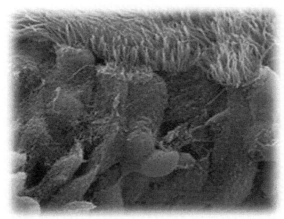

Many people are aware that dogs and some other animals have a much better sense of smell than humans. This is because the interiors of their noses have a much higher surface area, providing more of a space for smells to come into contact, with the cilia and therefore creating a larger filter for incoming smells.

Because humans have shortened noses and flat faces, rather than elongated snouts, they don't have the room for the extensive sensory membranes common to many animals. Intriguingly, many domesticated animals have shorter snouts than their wild relatives, suggesting that sense of smell may be one of the first senses to decrease with domestication.

There are cases in which olfactory cilia can be damaged or absent, impeding sense of smell and creating a condition called anosmia. While anosmia may sound like a minor inconvenience in humans, it can actually be quite dangerous, as the sense of smell is used to determine when food is going bad, whether gas leaks are present in an area, and to check for other signs of potential danger.

- Skin irritations
- Sensitive skin
- Sneezing
- Temperature
- Temperament
- Tick Poisoning

Tick Poisoning

Signs of tick poisoning can be detected if your dog is lethargic and has lost his appetite. They will be reticence to be active but the animal can be aroused to walk normally, although he may continue to refuse to eat. These pets may be developing some immunity.

If you catch the ticks early enough you can remove it and use the chicken broth as the convalescing food for a week or two.

Note: Gait is the pattern of movement of the limbs of animals, including humans, during locomotion over a solid substrate. Most animals use a variety of gaits, selecting gait based on speed, terrain, the need to maneuver, and energetic efficiency. Different animal species may use different gaits due to differences in anatomy that prevent use of certain gaits, or simply due to evolved innate preferences as a result of habitat differences.

However, if any signs of gait abnormality or vomiting/gagging or breathing difficulty develop-then these signs nearly always progress to the full paralysis syndrome. In other words, gait abnormalities, breathing difficulties, vomiting or gagging represent early signs rather than mild signs. Take advantage of the benefits of having anti-tick serum being given early- it is much more effective this way.

Whilst costs may be of concern, it is much less expensive to treat an early simple case of tick poisoning than it is to treat an advanced complicated case, in which pneumonia and heart failure have developed.

Tick Size

Once an adult female tick is engorged, to more than about 4 mm body width. The size of the tick has no bearing on severity if clinical signs are present. A 4 mm (body width) engorged tick is just as potentially deadly as a 10 mm engorged tick. Spray your yard with dilled peppermint and grow loads of peppermint to minimize the problem.

Eye Info

Also see the main heading for "**Eye Care**".
If eyelids are paralyzed (no blink reflex) the eye's corneal surface may need to be moistened. You can

use a sterile lubricant (e.g. Lacrilube K-Y), artificial tears, medical saline, or as a last resort even a drop of corn oil or olive oil (if the eye does not appear inflamed). Most antibiotic eye ointments are safe provided they do not contain any kind of cortisone.

What happens if my dog does not receive antiserum?

Dogs showing symptoms more than simply being lethargic or a loss of appetite have a "guarded" prognosis for survival if not given antiserum. From a general interpretation of the scientific literature "most" or "the vast majority" of dogs not receiving antiserum will die. In contrast to this, only about 5% of dogs receiving antiserum will die (and these are usually dogs that have received their antiserum at a late/advanced stage of tick poisoning). Dogs appear to be less likely to survive than cats.

Talking To Your Dog

Dog talk; If you take the time to listen, your dog and you will be able to understand each other very well. It is amazing what my dogs tell me. They make a different sound and perform different movements for everything they want to say to me.

You are their master and they treat you that way. However, they also rely on you to understand them when they are trying to tell you something. Tucker time is between 6 and 7 pm in our house and if I am late they tell me. Morning poo is between 6.30 and 7.30 am, and they want to go out at that time and they tell me. I love my dogs and they also love me and they let me know. When they are annoyed with me they also let me know. When I have been out somewhere and left them at home they jump for joy when I come through the door but they also bark with annoyance.

Defy Your Vet.

Ceasar Survived After Vet Wanted Him Put Down.

Yes, challenge your vet if you have a gut feeling that your dog is not ready to die. A few week before Ceasar was due to have his second vaccination he was attacked by three large dogs. After lots of cuddles, cleaning his wounds and giving him a complete check over he seemed fine. I also gave him some smelling salts for shock.

Like always him and Mark Antony cuddled up together in their bed. I was managing my daughters' hair and beauty salon at the time so I was able to take them to work with me and keep a close eye on them. Ceasar was booked in to have his second vaccination the following day but the Vet thought it best to give him a rest for a few days.

A few days later while on our morning walk, Ceasar collapsed. The main point I need to make here is how stupid I was. When you have a new puppy, you should not introduce them to other animals nor take them out into public places for a walk. It is important just like babies to wait until they are three months old and have had their vaccinations. When you break the rules you pay the price.

A few minutes after Ceasar collapsed he did a runny bloody poo. His eyes were glassy looking, his gums did not return to red when pressed, his pulse was 40 beats per minute. I rushed him to the Vet. The vet gave him an injection for the infection.

When I returned to the clinic to check on Ceasar that night he was sitting in a cage on newspaper filled with liquid that was a pale yellowish colour and lots of blood. The nurse said she would clean his cage. The vet said, your dog is going to die it would be kinder to put him down. I begged the vet to put him on a drip and the vet assured me he would yet tried to convince me it was probably a waste of money.

The next morning, I went to check on Ceasar again. He was still in the cage on bloody wet newspaper and the Vet had not given him a drip. When I asked why

Ceasar had not been put onto a drip the Vet made the excuse that it was pointless and that Ceasar was so ill he could not get the needle to go in. I begged the Vet to do something. He said, there was nothing more he could do and that I needed to allow time for Ceasar to settle down but he was sure I was going to loose, Ceasar. I then questioned the Vet about giving Ceasar an antibiotic injection.

Parvo if that was what Ceasar has is a virus and antibiotics would not actually help.

I went on to say
I know I do not have your knowledge but I feel sure that Ceasar needs fluids and electrolytes.

The vet responded
No he needs to be put down and released from his pain.

I immediately took Ceasar. The Vet followed me saying

You cannot take him he needs to stay here. He is very sick.

I through one hundred dollars at the Vet and kept walking. As fast as I could I took Ceasar to another vet and insisted he be put onto subcutaneous fluids for dogs. The new Vet agreed and I went to my car, I cried and prayed. A amazing feeling of peace came over me I felt that Ceasar was going to pull through.

Later that day I rang the Vet to organize a time for me to see Ceasar. When I returned for my visit, I was not allowed to see where Ceasar was being kept. I was ushered into a consultation room and they brought Ceasar into that room for our visit. They had his drip in place and although Ceasar was very feeble, his gums were a better colour and his blood returned comparatively quickly.

His pulse was still weak but had improved. They had also given him a dry shampoo. The only thing I was concerned about was how cold he felt. After our visit I went next door to the Pet shop and bought him a new coat. The Vet nurse was happy to put him in his new coat. Feeling relieved I did sleep better that night and did not go in the next morning for a morning visit. When I rang they said, there had been no change.

That night when I went in for my visit, Ceasar was a tiny bit more alert but he was freezing. So, when no one was looking I slipped out to where the animals are kept. The air-conditioner was very cold, back there. When I expressed my concerns to the nurse she said, there was nothing that could be done to change the temperature.

This rang alarm bells in my head. Immediately I spoke to the reception staff and said, I was going to take Ceasar home and asked if they could make up my account. The receptionist asked the Vet to talk with me.

He said, I could not take Ceasar home and that he was probably going to die and that it was best if he stay there so they could make his passing as comfortable for him as possible. When I insisted that I was going to take Ceasar home and would bring him in each day for a checkup the Vet became abusive. I overlooked his comments handed the receptionist two hundred and seventy dollars and said, please post me a receipt and what else I owe you can send me an account for. Then I turned around and walked out their door.

Well you are not going to believe what happen next.

I cannot remember all that the Vet said to me but it went something like this.

As I was walking with Ceasar in my arms the vet comes up behind me and calls me a bloody idiot as he push me in the small of my back. I fell to my knees with one elbow on the ground and Ceasar still held in my other arm. As I was trying to get up the Vet was yelling at me saying he was going to get the police and he tried to snatch Ceasar from me.

He went on to say we are not a charity your dog has been well cared for and you need to pay for my service.

With both arms around Ceasar I gained my footing, also holding the drip and my handbag, I looked the Vet straight in the eye and said:-

Step back, do not touch me or my dog, send me a bill. Now step back.

I cannot remember what he was yelling at me about as he walked away. But, I got into my car with Ceasar and was so shaken-up by the entire ordeal I burst into tears.

Well the good news is Ceasar is still here, alive and well, It is now nine years later. Yes, I should have waited for them to make-up my account but Ceasar was freezing and I needed to get him home. As it turned out, I only needed to give the vet another $35 dollars.

Administering Treatment To Ceasar.

I checked with the Washington State University on how to care for Caesars drip. You can go to their pet health section on the internet and they give you step by step instructions with lots of step by step photographs on administering subcutaneous fluids.

http://www.vetmed.wsu.edu/outreach/Pet-Health-Topics/categories

While you're on their site please make a small donation.

Well thanks to WSU and my Aromatherapy training, I had no trouble with Ceasars drip. I administered him chicken broth with a eye dropper every hour, massaged him several times a day with Aromatherapy oils and he did not die.

I have never told anyone about my ordeal with both the Veterinary surgeons and now everyone that reads this book will know. True love really does over come and conquer all.

Urination

Dogs cannot express themselves through words; it is the duty of a dog owner, to make sure that the pet enjoys the best of health. It is important to be on a lookout for signs of poor health.

The colour of the urine can sometimes provide valuable insights on the health of your dog. If the dog's urine is dark yellow in colour and also has a strong odor, the best thing to do is to take your dog to a vet.

<hr>

Causes

The colour of the urine is an indicator of the kidney function. Under normal circumstances, the urine must not be concentrated and the colour of the urine must be light yellow.

Dehydration: Dark yellow urine may be indicative of dehydration. If left untreated, an excessive loss of electrolytes or body fluids can even cause an organ failure. Fluid loss could take place in hot weather, or may also occur due to vomiting or diarrhea.

If fluid loss that takes place due to breathing, panting, urination or evaporation through the feet or body, if not compensated, the body tries to retain fluids and thus, the urine may become concentrated.

Urine colour may change from pale yellow to dark yellow under such circumstances. Lethargy, loss of appetite, sunken eyes, dry mouth, dark yellow urine with strong odor or too little urine are some of the symptoms that a dehydrated dog may exhibit.

Ailments: Formation of kidney stones or bladder stones could also occur as a result of dehydration. If the dog is not drinking enough water, the urine would become concentrated, and the minerals in urine may crystallize to form hard stone-like deposits. These stones can obstruct the passage of urine and cause painful urination. Besides bladder problems or kidney stones, liver problems could also be responsible for the change in the colour of your pet's urine.

Jaundice is one such condition that may be responsible for the change in the colour of urine from pale yellow to dark yellow. Pancreas problems, diabetes, urinary tract infection or hemolytic anemia also figure in the list of ailments that may affect the urine odor as well as urine colour. Old dogs who have been diagnosed with an ailment, may have to be administered certain drugs. The dark yellow urine may be due to use of supplements or drugs.

Dog Food: Just like us, animals are also likely to suffer from health problems if their diet is not providing them with the required nutrients. Naturally, it is essential that you identify the brands that are known for providing good quality dog food. This will ensure your pet is not ingesting food that may contain toxins or additives. If your pet doesn't get healthy food, there is a great risk of your dog suffering from health problems, which in turn, may give rise to various distressing symptoms.

Never give your dog table scraps and biscuits that you like to eat.

Shampoo For Pets

Make Our Own Pet Shampoo.

Buy some pure soap from the supermarket. You will find pure soap in the same section as the laundry detergents.

- Grate one to two bars of the pure soap.
- Place soap in a large mixing bowl

Add:-
- One and a half liters of boiling water
- One teaspoon of olive oil
- One tablespoon of vinegar
- Two drops of rose geranium
- Six drops of chamomile.

Now mix or blend until you have smooth paste.
Place this mix into a large jar. Wrap paper around the jar to keep the contents away from light. Store the shampoo in a cool dark place.

This shampoo can be used on all pets and the family. Shelf life is six months.

You can place half the mixture into a food safe container and keep in the freezer but be sure to place a tag on the container stating that it is shampoo.

Teeth

Yes, I know that most of you think giving your dog raw beef and lamb bones to chew on will clean their teeth. You are right of cause, but bones alone will not do. You also need to clean their teeth.

As this book is about helping you to reduce your vet bills, you need to be diligent in keeping your dogs teeth clean.

Periodontal disease is one of the most common problems
The first is gingivitis, a reversible inflammation of the gums.
The second is periodontitis, an inflammation of the deeper structures supporting the teeth.

Gingivitis

Gingivitis develops when bacteria build up between the teeth and gums, leading to irritation, inflammation, and bleeding. The edges of healthy gums fit tightly around the teeth. In a dog with gingivitis, rough dental calculus builds up in an irregular fashion along the gum line, producing points at which the gum is forced away from the teeth. This creates small pockets that trap food and bacteria. In time, the gums become infected.

Dental calculus (also called tartar) is composed of calcium salts, food particles, bacteria, and other organic material. It is yellow-brown and soft when first deposited.

At the soft stage, it is called plaque. The plaque quickly hardens into calculus. Calculus collects on all tooth surfaces, but is found - in the greatest amounts on the cheek side of the upper premolars and molars.

This buildup of calculus on the teeth is the primary cause of gum inflammation. This occurs to some extent in all dogs over the age of 2. Certain breeds, such as Poodles, and smaller dogs seem to form calculus more readily.

Dogs that eat dry kibble and chew on bones or dog biscuits have less calculus buildup than dogs that eat only soft, canned foods.

A characteristic sign of gingivitis is bad breath. The halitosis may have been present for some time-even accepted as normal. The gums appear red and swollen, and bleed easily when touched. Pressing on the gums may cause pus to ooze from the gum line.

Treatment: Treatment is directed toward preventing gingivitis from progressing to periodontitis and delaying the progress of periodontitis once it is established.

The teeth should be, professionally cleaned, scaled, and polished to remove all plaque and calculus. Many veterinarians now use ultrasonic dental units, similar to the ones used on people, for cleaning dogs' teeth. For optimum results, the dog should be heavily sedated or given a general anesthetic.

The cleaning should be followed with a regular regimen of home oral care.

Periodontitis

Periodontitis develops as a continuation of gingivitis. The teeth are held in their bony sockets by a substance called cementum and a specialized connective tissue called, the periodontal membrane. As the gum infection attacks the cementum and periodontal membrane (see above the figure Structure of a Tooth), the roots become infected, the teeth begin to loosen, and eventually they detach. This is a painful process. Although the dog's appetite is good, she may sit by her food dish, eat reluctantly, and drop food from her mouth.

Drooling is common. A root abscess can rupture into the maxillary sinus or nasal cavity, producing a purulent unilateral
nasal discharge, an oral-nasal fistula or a swelling below the eye.

Treatment: The teeth should be professionally cleaned, as described for gingivitis. Severe infections may necessitate removing a portion of the diseased gum (a procedure called gingivectomy). In a dog with advanced periodontitis, it may be necessary to extract some or all of the teeth before healing can begin.

Once the gums are healed, a dog without teeth is able to eat surprisingly well. Antibiotics are given for one to three weeks, depending on the severity of the disease.

Aftercare at home involves rinsing the mouth with 0.2 percent chlorhexidine solution (Peridex or Nolvadent) once or twice a day. Soak a cotton ball and gently swab the gums and teeth, or use a plastic syringe and squirt the antiseptic directly onto the teeth and gums. You can also brush the dog's teeth with a dog tooth brush and a toothpaste made especially for dogs that contains chlorhexidine.

Massage the gums with your finger, a piece of linen, or a soft gauze pad, using a gentle circular motion, while pressing on the outside surface of the gums. Continue the mouth washes and massages until the gums are healthy. I suggest weekly for a few weeks then once a month thereafter. Feed a soft diet consisting of canned dog food mixed with water to make a mush. Once healing is complete, switch to a good home dental program.

A product called Stomadhex, available through your veterinarian, may prove to be an effective substitute for the aftercare just described. Stomadhex is a small adhesive patch that sticks to mucous membranes. The patch is applied to the inside surface of the upper lip. It stays in place for several hours and slowly releases chlorhexidine and a vitamin called nicotinamide that promotes oral hygiene. The sustained release delivery system helps to prevent dental plaque and tartar and aids in controlling bad breath. The patch is applied daily for 10 days following a dental procedure, or as recommended by your veterinarian.

Vaccination

See heading **"Immunization"**

Vomiting

Dogs devour grass with a view to bring on vomiting and get rid of any noxious substance that they might have consumed. Check the vomit if there is a small parcel of undigested grass in the pile then your dog knows he is not well and has tried to fix the problem himself. If the vomiting lasts for more than a day you need to go to the Vet.

Walking

It is very important to ofter allow your dog to roam free. Keeping them on a lead all the time causes pscological problems. Find a fenced park and allow them to play freely at least four times a week.

The bacteria that cause tetanus are found in soil and animal feces. So pick up your dogs poo as quickly as you can and place in a bag then in the garbage bin. It is very important to walk your dog twice a day. Take your dog on his lead for his daily walk and pick up his poo. A small walk around the block is sufficient most days.

Several times a week he needs to go some-where he can run free.

Take liver treats with you in your pocket. Every few minutes call him back to you and give him a treat and tell him he is a good dog. If his playing happily with other dogs leave him be until the other dogs and their owners start to walk off. I find if I say "bye" and start to walk in the direction of my car or where I want them to walk. They soon leave the other dogs and follow me.

I also say "bye" every time I leave the house to go somewhere without them. They soon understand that is the word I say when I am going somewhere without them. They are like children when you say bye sweet heart I have to go to the shops I will be back soon. Children start to cry and run and hold you tight. Dogs and children do not like you to go anywhere without them.

If you had to look at your fences while on your knees every day how would you feel? I am sure you would soon become very bored and depressed.

Sometimes when my dogs are playing with other dogs I walk in the opposite direction this causes them to be a little uncertain about me. This is a good thing as it gives you a bit more control. I also change the amount of time we stay at the free run area and the direction I walk. Up until your dog is about four years of age they can become a bit too sure of you and wonder off.

They follow the smells of other dogs and can get them self lost. From four years of age onwards their sense of direction gets better and even if they do wonder off they can find their way home. This is providing they do not meet with the dog ranger or someone that thinks this dog has been, abandoned.

If you have been taking them for long walks along the footpath through your town and only crossing at the traffic lights or foot crossings that is what they will do when on their own.

It is very cruel to keep a dog on a tight lead every day. He wants to smell things close up that he can sense in the distance.

It is also very cruel to keep him in the yard all day every day smelling the same smells seeing the same fence day in and day out.

Weight Changes

It is important to know how much your dog weighs. Most vets will allow you to pop in a few times a year to have your dog weighed. Then when his sick you will know if he has lost weight. If he has you can inform the vet.

Whinging Whining

Ceasar never does either but my other dog Mark Antony does both. Mark Antony is a very vocal dog. If he wants to go outside and I have locked the door he has a whinge at me from a distance and gives me a long hard stare. If I have been talking to my friends - too long he has another kind of whinge. Went his in pain there is another type of whining. He has a few different kinds of barks to tell me things and a jumping run around in circle action for I need a walk. Ceasar gets his message across but in a quite passive way.

Ceasar stands near the refrigerator when his hungry and puts his head forward and looks at me long and hard until I feed him.

It is important to take notice of them because they will convey their needs to you in their own special way.

Dog Whining just like any other dog behavior, must be understood before it can be dealt with. The best dog training comes from understanding and knowing your dog.

Whining is one of four basic ways that a dog communicates vocally. Barking, growling, and howling are the other three ways.

A dog whines when he is in distress or when he is looking for attention. Whining when in distress is a natural thing and should not be discouraged. You should want to know when your dog is in distress. Whining for attention on the other hand is something that you should want to curb.

There are three basic ways you can respond to your dog's whining:

1. To ignore your dog's whining completely is not the right choice because your dog will think that you do not care. There is also some chance that your dog is whining for a real reason like a sickness. You should not ignore your dog's whining.

2. Immediately, come to your dog every time he whines even the slightest bit. I try to work out what he wants and attend to the issue.

3. You will soon understand if he is whining for attention. When this is the case, I tell him to go outside.

The different reasons why your dog may be whining:

1. Anxiety Your dog may be experiencing separation anxiety when you leave him alone. One way to solve this problem is to leave him alone for longer and longer periods of time, but only very gradually. This way he gets used to spending more and more time alone rather than, all of a sudden having to spend very long times alone.

2. Pain If your dog is whining because he or she is in pain then you will want to find out what is wrong with your dog and you may want to take him to the vet.

3. Knots in his hair close to the skin can cause a lot of pain. The dog will try to remove the knots by chewing them out, but that is not always possible for him. When you are brushing, your dog do not tag at the knots that hurts and causes internal burses. Cut the knots out.

4.   Attention Seeking. This is the reason that most needs to be nipped in the bud. You cannot allow your dog to get your attention every time he whines. You have to check at first to make sure that he is ok but then you may want to let him realize that you are not going pamper him every time he whines.

Worms

As you would know, worms are a real killer. It is important to give them the big heave-ho.

Signs telling you that your dog has worms

Common symptoms to watch out for

Since your dog can't speak English well, you need to be diligent in watching out for your dog and noticing any unusual signs. Here are some common ways to tell if your dog has worms.

Visible worms or eggs in fecal matter - This is the most common way to confirm that your dog has worms. However, not all kinds of worms are visible in fecal matter to the naked eye.

Visible worms in fur, or area around dog's rear - Tapeworms, in particular, may appear as small moving segments, which later dry out to resemble grains of rice.

Scratching or rubbing of rear on the ground or against furniture - if your dog shows signs of itchiness around the rear, it may be irritated by worms in the area.
However, this could also be due to problems with glands unrelated to worms.

Vomiting with visible worms - if your dog has worms, you may also see them in your dog's vomit.
 Bloated stomach or belly - This is another common symptom of worms, often seen in puppies who receive worms from their mother.

Weakness, increased appetite, constant hunger, weight loss - If your dog has worms, the worms are stealing your dog's nutrition. Your dog may be weak or constantly hungry, and in severe cases, may be losing weight.

Diarrhea, particularly with blood in it.

Why Your Dog Might Have Worms

Newly born puppies always have worms - roundworm eggs can form cysts in adult dogs that remain dormant. These eggs CANNOT be removed by medication.

When a female dog is pregnant, these dormant eggs will activate and infect the puppies. The mother's milk can also pass roundworms to puppies.

Contact with infected dirt - roundworm eggs and hookworm larvae can reside in dirt. If your dog came in contact with infected dirt, your dog may get worms.

Fleas - young tapeworms can reside in fleas. If your dog swallows fleas while grooming, your dog will ingest tapeworms and be infected.

Hunting or eating wildlife - wild animals may carry worms, including tapeworms residing in fleas on wild animals. If your dog hunts or eats wildlife, your dog may swallow worms.

How do you know if your dog has something besides worms?

A Dog Owner's Guide To Diagnosis And Treatment

Some of the symptoms for worms, such as stomach irritation, can be confused with other health problems. Keeping your dog healthy means you need to be alert to - Warning signs, for a range or problems, not just worms. You can always bring your dog to the veterinarian, but the first line of defense, is YOU, the dog owner at HOME, not the veterinarian's office.

In addition, medication can have side effects, and some dogs react poorly to medicines prescribed by the veterinarian. Even after you visit the veterinarian, you need to carefully observe your dog and know when there is another problem.

If you are interested in learning how to take care of your dog's health from home, and what health problems to look out for, I recommend that you devote some time to learning about dog health issues. This means a lot of reading, at least in the beginning! You can ask your veterinarian to recommend literature. Easy-to-read, but reputable, magazines are also a great source of health information.

Symptoms and risks for worm infections

Roundworms

Roundworms - roundworms can grow up to half a foot in length and live in the intestines. They should be visible as small noodle-like bits in fecal/faeces (poo) matter and cause swollen bellies. Roundworms are a big problem with puppies.

Because roundworms can enter your dog's body in many different ways, it is essential to keep your dog's living area clean, remove feces Roundworm in dog's intestineregularly, and, if possible, prevent your dog from eating wild animals that may carry roundworms.

To get rid of roundworms that are passed from the mother dog, puppies should be treated at 2, 4, 6, and 8 weeks of age and then receive a preventive treatment monthly. Fecal (stool) examinations should be conducted 2 to 4 times during the first year of life and 1 or 2 times each year in adults. Nursing mothers should be kept on monthly preventive and treated along with their puppies to decrease the risk of transmission.

Many heartworm preventives also control roundworms. Ask your veterinarian about prevention and treatment choices that are appropriate for your dog.

Can Humans Be Harmed By Roundworms?

Roundworms do pose a significant risk to humans. Contact with contaminated soil or dog feces can result in human ingestion and infection. Roundworm eggs may accumulate in significant numbers in the soil where pets deposit feces. Once infected, the worms can cause eye, lung, heart and neurologic signs in people.

Children should not be allowed to play where animals have passed feces. Individuals who have direct contact with soil that may have been contaminated by cat or dog feces should wear gloves or wash their hands immediately.

Hookworms

Hookworms - hookworms are thin, small worms that "bite" or "hook" into the intestinal wall. They are not always visible by eye, which means a microscope examination is needed to observe eggs in fecal matter. Hookworms can cause bleeding because of their biting, which results in bloody stools or anemia.

Tapeworms

Tapeworms - tapeworms are flat, long worms that live in the intestines. Segments of the tapeworm breaking off are visible to the naked eye as rice-like grains after drying out. They are look like rice grains in your dogs poo.

Heartworms

Heart worms can be controlled once a year with a heart worm injection. This can be arranged at your local veterinary clinic. But, you can give your dog tablets. Talk with the local Pet Shop.

Heartworms are one of the most dangerous worms because they cannot easily, be detected. Heartworms, can be spread by mosquitoes.

Heartworms damage the heart muscle and require a blood test to detect. Heart damage can be fatal, and you will only see other symptoms such as weakness or dull fur after heart damage has already occurred. It is absolutely necessary to keep your dog on a heartworm preventive medicine.

Whipworms

Whipworms are thin, thread like worms living in the large intestine. Adults may be visible by the naked eye, but fecal matter does not contain many worms, so they may be difficult to detect. A microscope examination of several fecal samples may be necessary to detect them. Whipworms are one of the most difficult worms to eliminate, but they are treatable.

How to treat your dog for worms.

Do not wait till you think your dog has worms. Safe and effective treatments are readily available.

For the most common types of worms, including heartworms, roundworms, hookworms, and tapeworms, there are all-in-one medications for your dog in flavored chewable tablets.

For example, tablets are useful for treating all four of these conditions and includes three active ingredients: ivermectin to prevent heartworm, pyrantel pamoate to treat roundworms and hookworms, and praziquantel to treat tapeworms.

Since this kind of medication covers all the major worm types, it is a very convenient multi-purpose medication for the average dog owner. You need to determine the correct dosage based on your dog's weight, but most of these medications require one tablet a month. Some flea control treatments cover the worms as well.

Warnings about worm medications.

It is important to note that some tablets only deal with a few worm types. Most medications in supermarkets sell packs that do not cover tapeworms and heartworms. Personally, I like pet stores for the purchase of worm medications. The staff, are usually well trained and happy to answer your questions without charging you a fee.

As for all the other worms give your dog a worm tablet as per the instructions on the pack. I do not like the chewable tablets as the dog may spit some of it out when you are not looking. I buy the type of tablet that you can crush up and put into their food.

I do not give them any food during the day that I am going to worm them. This way they are very hungry when I do feed them about an hour or more later, than their usual nightly feed time. They will be able to smell the tablet so they need to be very hungry when you put their food in front of them. Put less food in the bowl than usual. This way you are sure they eat it all and get the tablet into their system.

Then give them some more food.

When they finish eating give them a treat. That way they will come to know that on the night their food smells odd, they get rewards. It is best to give then a casserole style meal the night you are administering their tablet.

Many people are good at giving medications to dogs but my two little darlings can smell that tablet and run under my bed and will not come out.

If you are able to, you can hold the underside of their mouth at the same time put the tablet in the back of their mouth and then quickly hold their mouth shut. They do not like this method but, it is a quick way to get the job done.

How Often To Treat The Dog For Worms

There are recommendations on the worm tablet packets. If my dogs have had a bout of fleas then I keep the worming program to the suggested intervals on the pack.

If they have not had any fleas for a while, I give them a break from worming medications for about two months then I retreat them. I am not recommending you do this.

As an Aromatherapist, with all the other natural therapies I administer, I like to give their system a break from chemicals.

Heartworms on the other hand are a problem that cannot be detected until it is too late. That is why I have them vaccinated every twelve months by the Vet. When it is not financially possible for you to have them vaccinated then you will need to keep the heartworm tables administered to your dog every six weeks.

Other Books By
Robyna Smith-Keys

Healing Manuals

Foolproof Aromatherapy

Essential oils can heal, sooth and energize. Learn how to mix. When not to use and all the benefits for hundreds of ailments listed in alphabetical order. User friendly.

The Antique Healer

This is a much large Aromatherapy book with photos and more healings. Also contains wise old women's remedies.

Organic Cancer Cure (Free)

I Was Not Ready To Lose My Mother. My mother had a few weeks to live. Her Cancer was very aggressive. I set her up on a healing program of juices, essential oils and herbs. This was all working until she stopped the program. It also has a lovely storey about her life. Married at age 16 until her Passover at 83 years of age.

Natural Organic Skincare Recipes (eBook)

Organic Skincare

Both these books teach you how to mix your own healing recipes with essential oils. They explain the importance of electronic facials and the cheapest way to have a facial.

Dog Care & DIY Organic Medications {EBook} Plus in Print

There are times you cannot afford a Vet. We also explore the worm tablets and their effects. A very handy book, for all dog lovers.

How To Training Manuals.

Body Piercing Basics

All the main points on body piercing.

Anatomy For Body Piercers

All Body Piercers should understand the body and how it works this is a wonderful tool for any Body Piercer.

An Angel For Cosmetic Tattooists

A helping hand for a cosmetic tattooist.

Cosmetic Tattoo Permanent Makeup Micro-pigmentation Training Manual

A step by step training manual. You could actually teach yourself the trade as this book is so well written.

Eyelash Extensions Grafted Lashes Training Manual
Step by step instructions with video tutorials. Also cover false eyelashes and party lashes.

Eyebrows Shaping And Tinting To Suit Face Shapes
Step by step instructions with video tutorials on eyebrow shaping, eyelash and brow tinting

.

Face & Body Waxing Cosmetology Hair Removal Training Manual
With step by step instruction. Types of wax and their appropriate use for each body part. Plus contraindications.

Hair Extensions Training Manual
Learn to create hair wefts, weaves, braids, wax in, and clip in Hair Extensions. There are videos to watch in the eBook.

Supernatural Books:-

Numerology Basics
Describes your personal year and lessons to learn each year. Your personality and what type of work best suits your personality. This book is brief and to the point. This book is brief and to the point.

Numerology Folklore

Describes your personal year and lessons to learn each year. Your personality and what type of work best suits your personality. How to Journal your life and make the big changes.

Spell Folklore

A great book on how to do some positive affirmations also called spells.

Tarot Scrolls 0-22

Ask a question open a page and an inspiring answer will be there for you to read.

Positive Thinking

Ba Ha Ha Happy

Loaded with affirmations and verses for you to read each day to keep you sane. I loved writing this book. Evan if no one else ever reads it, what I affirmed to myself during the process of trying to think about real life situation and how best to handle them, has been a tattoo in my mind.

Mind Blossoms

How to lift your thoughts in a positive way.

Positive Spiritual Affirmations

A smaller version of Ba Ha Ha Happy!

Children's Books:-

Romeo and Juliette Keep Mark Antony

A wonderful storey about a puppy born on a boat. His white cute and fluffy. True storey with a dash of magic added.

Mark Antony Marries Lizy and Has Puppies

Loaded with photos of all the dogs and the new born puppies. A true story with a dash of fantasy added.

Contact Robyna at
email; beautyschoolbooks@gmail.com
Facebook:
https://www.facebook.com/AromatherapyAndBeautySchoolBooks/

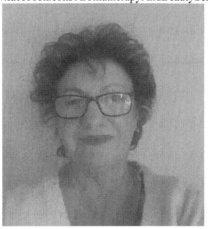

Good luck everyone I pray this DIY animal care will assist you to save some money and care for your pet, in a loving caring manner and save you and your pet from anxious moments. I am by no means any kind of author but I have been very broke at times in my life when my pets needed help. I trust that this book will help someone else and their pet live longer. All too often people think about either giving up their pet or having him/her put to sleep because of the cost of healing their pet.

###

81200625R00128

Made in the USA
Middletown, DE
21 July 2018